Urologic Trauma and Reconstruction

Editors

ALLEN F. MOREY
STEVEN J. HUDAK

UROLOGIC CLINICS
OF NORTH AMERICA

www.urologic.theclinics.com

Consulting Editor
SAMIR S. TANEJA

August 2013 • Volume 40 • Number 3

ELSEVIER

1600 John F. Kennedy Boulevard • Suite 1800 • Philadelphia, Pennsylvania, 19103-2899

http://www.theclinics.com

UROLOGIC CLINICS OF NORTH AMERICA Volume 40, Number 3
August 2013 ISSN 0094-0143, ISBN-13: 978-0-323-18618-6

Editor: Stephanie Donley

Urologic Clinics of North America (ISSN 0094-0143) is published quarterly by Elsevier Inc., 360 Park Avenue South, New York, N 10010-1710. Months of issue are February, May, August, and November. Business and Editorial Offices: 1600 John F. Kenned Blvd., Suite 1800, Philadelphia, PA 19103-2899. Periodicals postage paid at New York, NY and additional mailing offices. Sub scription prices are $339.00 per year (US individuals), $583.00 per year (US institutions), $396.00 per year (Canadian individuals $713.00 per year (Canadian institutions), $492.00 per year (foreign individuals), and $713.00 per year (foreign institutions). Foreig air speed delivery is included in all *Clinics* subscription prices. All prices are subject to change without notice. **POSTMASTEF** Send address changes to *Urologic Clinics of North America*, Elsevier Health Sciences Division, Subscription Customer Service 3251 Riverport Lane, Maryland Heights, MO 63043. Customer Service: 1-800-654-2452 (US). From outside the Unite States, call 1-314-447-8871. Fax: 1-314-447-8029. E-mail: JournalsCustomerServiceusa@elsevier.com (for print support) an JournalsOnlineSupport-usa@elsevier.com (for online support).

Reprints. For copies of 100 or more, of articles in this publication, please contact the Commercial Reprints Department, Elsevie Inc., 360 Park Avenue South, New York, New York 10010-1710. Tel.: 212-633-3813; Fax: 212-462-1935; E-mail: reprints@ elsevier.com.

Urologic Clinics of North America is covered in MEDLINE/PubMed (*Index Medicus*), *Excerpta Medica, Current Contents Clinical Medicine, Science Citation Index,* and *ISI/BIOMED.*

Printed and bound by CPI Group (UK) Ltd, Croydon, CR0 4YY

Transferred to digital print 2013

Contributors

CONSULTING EDITOR

SAMIR S. TANEJA, MD
The James M. Neissa and Janet Riha Neissa
Professor of Urologic Oncology, Professor of
Urology and Radiology, Director, Division of
Urologic Oncology, Co-Director, Smilow
Comprehensive Prostate Cancer Center,
Department of Urology, NYU Langone Medical
Center, New York, New York

EDITORS

ALLEN F. MOREY, MD
Professor, Department of Urology,
UT Southwestern Medical Center, Dallas,
Texas

STEVEN J. HUDAK, MD
Staff Urologist, Department of Surgery,
Urology Section, San Antonio Military Medical
Center, Fort Sam Houston; Clinical Assistant
Professor, Department of Urology, University
of Texas Health Science Center, San Antonio,
Texas

AUTHORS

NATHANIEL K. BALLEK, MD
Fellow Genitourinary Reconstruction,
Department of Urology, Northwestern
University Feinberg School of Medicine,
Chicago, Illinois

STEVEN B. BRANDES, MD
Division of Urologic Surgery, Washington
University School of Medicine, St Louis, Missouri

WILLIAM O. BRANT, MD, FACS
Department of Surgery, The Center for
Reconstructive Urology and Men's Health,
University of Utah, Salt Lake City, Utah

BENJAMIN N. BREYER, MD, MAS
Assistant Professor, Department of Urology,
University of California, San Francisco,
California

JOSHUA A. BROGHAMMER, MD, FACS
Department of Urology, University of Kansas
Medical Center, Kansas City, Kansas

ANDREW J. CHANG, MD
Division of Urologic Surgery, Washington
University School of Medicine, St Louis,
Missouri

MICHAEL COBURN, MD, FACS
Professor and Chairman, Scott Department
of Urology, Baylor College of Medicine,
Houston, Texas

DAVID A. DUCHENE, MD, FACS
Associate Professor, Department of
Urology, Director of Minimally Invasive
Surgery and Kidney Stone Disease,
University of Kansas Medical Center,
Kansas City, Kansas

DANIEL D. DUGI III, MD
Assistant Professor, Department of Urology,
Oregon Health and Sciences University,
Portland, Oregon

JOEL GELMAN, MD
Clinical Professor of Urology, Department of
Urology, Director, Center for Reconstructive
Urology, University of California Irvine Medical
Center, Orange, California

CHRISTOPHER M. GONZALEZ, MD, MBA
Professor of Urology, Director of Genitourinary
Reconstruction, Department of Urology,
Northwestern University Feinberg School of
Medicine, Chicago, Illinois

STEVEN J. HUDAK, MD
Staff Urologist, Department of Surgery,
Urology Section, San Antonio Military Medical
Center, Fort Sam Houston; Clinical Assistant
Professor, Department of Urology, University
of Texas Health Science Center, San Antonio,
Texas

RICHARD B. KNIGHT, MD
Urology Resident, Department of Urology,
San Antonio Uniformed Services Health
Education Consortium, Fort Sam Houston,
Texas

LAURA LEDDY, MD
Department of Urology, Harborview Medical
Center, University of Washington School of
Medicine, Seattle, Washington

RYAN MAUCK, MD
Department of Urology, UT Southwestern
Medical Center, Dallas, Texas

JAMES B. McGEADY, MD
Urologic Trauma and Reconstructive Fellow,
Department of Urology, University of California,
San Francisco, California

ALLEN F. MOREY, MD
Professor, Department of Urology,
UT Southwestern Medical Center, Dallas,
Texas

JEREMY B. MYERS, MD, FACS
Department of Surgery, The Center for
Reconstructive Urology and Men's Health,
University of Utah, Salt Lake City, Utah

DANIEL RAMIREZ, MD
Department of Urology, UT Southwestern
Medical Center, Dallas, Texas

JAY SIMHAN, MD
Department of Urology, UT Southwestern
Medical Center, Dallas, Texas

THOMAS G. SMITH III, MD, FACS
Assistant Professor, Scott Department of
Urology, Baylor College of Medicine, Houston,
Texas

TIMOTHY J. TAUSCH, MD
Chief Resident, Madigan Army Medical Center,
Tacoma, Washington

HEMA J. THAKAR, MD
Assistant Professor, Division of Plastic and
Reconstructive Surgery, Department of
Surgery, Oregon Health and Sciences
University, Portland, Oregon

BRYAN VOELZKE, MD
Department of Urology, Harborview Medical
Center, University of Washington School of
Medicine, Seattle, Washington

HUNTER WESSELLS, MD
Department of Urology, Harborview Medical
Center, University of Washington School of
Medicine, Seattle, Washington

ANDREW P. WINDSPERGER, MD
Department of Urology, University of Kansas
Medical Center, Kansas City, Kansas

LEE C. ZHAO, MD
Fellow in Trauma, Reconstruction and
Prosthetics, Department of Urology,
UT Southwestern Medical Center, Dallas,
Texas

Contents

> This article reviews recent publications evaluating the current epidemiology of urologic trauma. The authors briefly explain databases that have been recently used to study this patient population and then discuss each genitourinary organ individually, utilizing the most relevant and up-to-date information published for each one. The conclusion of the article briefly discusses possible future research and development areas pertaining to the topic.

> With the advent of advanced trauma critical care, and precise methods of assessing renal trauma with computed tomography, most patients with high-grade renal trauma can be managed conservatively. Some patients, however, do not do well with conservative management. This article evaluates specific radiographic characteristics that have recently been associated with intervention for renal hemorrhage after trauma.

> This article discusses the evaluation and management of genitourinary system trauma in the critically injured patient. Injuries to any of the organs in the genitourinary system can be managed with a damage control strategy. Often, there is little or no preoperative imaging or injury staging, and these injuries are diagnosed intraoperatively. Finally, specific management strategies of renal, ureteral, bladder, urethral, and genital injuries are discussed.

> This article presents a review of the literature regarding surgical techniques and outcomes for reconstruction of strictures involving the upper ureter. The preoperative assessment for proximal ureteral stricture is briefly reviewed, followed by a discussion of ureteroureterostomy, transureteroureterostomy, ureterocalicostomy, bladder flaps, downward nephropexy, bowel interposition grafts, onlay or tubular grafting, renal autotransplantation, and nephrectomy. The future direction for reconstruction of the proximal ureter is proposed.

Distal ureteral reconstruction is increasingly being performed by minimally-invasive surgical techniques. The robotic surgical platform provides an additional modality for repairing distal ureteral defects with the associated benefits of a minimally-invasive approach. This article reviews and describes the technical aspects of robotic distal ureteral reconstruction. In addition to discussion of the operative technique, factors such as patient selection, preoperative and postoperative evaluation, and published outcomes are addressed.

Bladder neck contracture is a relatively uncommon but well-described complication after the surgical treatment of prostate cancer. Although numerous treatments have been described as an initial management strategy for patients with this condition, the management of refractory cases remains highly variable. This article evaluates various therapeutic maneuvers used for the treatment of refractory bladder neck contracture and further describes the preliminary results of an endoscopic balloon dilation with concomitant deep traunsurethral incision procedure. Short- and long-term management algorithms for patients with recurrent bladder neck contractures are reviewed.

This article provides an overview of the open surgical management of posterior urethral disruption injuries. The discussion includes the evaluation of the patient before surgery with a focus on urethral imaging and details of posterior urethroplasty surgical technique.

This article reviews the history, indications, technique, complications, and outcomes of primary urethral realignment of pelvic fracture urethral injuries. In clinically stable patients, an attempt at endoscopic urethral realignment is appropriate and may result in long-term urethral patency. However, long term follow up is necessary due to elevated rates of delayed stricture formation requiring endoscopic or surgical repair.

Reoperative urethroplasty is complicated by increased urethral and periurethral scar and the frequent persistence of comorbid conditions that caused the original failure. Nevertheless, by experienced clinicians, reoperative urethral reconstruction can be completed with success rates comparable with those of primary urethroplasty.

PROGRAM OBJECTIVE
The goal of Urologic Clinics of North America is to keep practicing urologists and urology residents up to date with current clinical practice in urology by providing timely articles reviewing the state of the art in patient care.

TARGET AUDIENCE
Practicing urologists, urology residents and other health care professionals practicing in the discipline of urology.

LEARNING OBJECTIVES
Upon completion of this activity, participants will be able to:
1. Review reconstruction of traumatic and reoperative anterior urethral strictures via excisional techniques as well as reconstruction of radiation-induced injuries of the lower urinary tract.
2. Discuss damage control maneuvers for urologic trauma.
3. Recognize advances in diagnosis and management of genital injuries.

ACCREDITATION
The Elsevier Office of Continuing Medical Education (EOCME) is accredited by the Accreditation Council for Continuing Medical Education (ACCME) to provide continuing medical education for physicians.

The EOCME designates this enduring material for a maximum of 15 *AMA PRA Category 1 Credit*(s)™. Physicians should claim only the credit commensurate with the extent of their participation in the activity.

All other health care professionals requesting continuing education credit for this enduring material will be issued a certificate of participation.

DISCLOSURE OF CONFLICTS OF INTEREST
The EOCME assesses conflict of interest with its instructors, faculty, planners, and other individuals who are in a position to control the content of CME activities. All relevant conflicts of interest that are identified are thoroughly vetted by EOCME for fair balance, scientific objectivity, and patient care recommendations. EOCME is committed to providing its learners with CME activities that promote improvements or quality in healthcare and not a specific proprietary business or a commercial interest.

The planning committee, staff, authors and editors listed below have identified no financial relationships or relationships to products or devices they or their spouse/life partner have with commercial interest related to the content of this CME activity:
Nathaniel K. Ballek, MD; Steven B. Brandes, MD; William O. Brant, MD, FACS; Benjamin N. Breyer, MD, MAS; Joshua A. Broghammer, MD, FACS; Andrew J. Chang, MD; Michael Coburn, MD; Nicole Congleton; Stephanie Donley; David A. Duchene, MD; Daniel D. Dugi III, MD; Joel Gelman, MD; Christopher M. Gonzalez, MD; Steven J. Hudak, MD; Richard B. Knight, MD; Indu Kumari; Sandy Lavery; Laura Leddy, MD; Ryan Mauck, MD; James B. McGeady, MD; Jill McNair; Jeremy B. Myers, MD; Daniel Ramirez, MD; Jay Simhan, MD; Thomas G. Smith III, MD, FACS; Timothy J. Tausch, MD, MS; Hema J. Thakar, MD; Bryan Voelzke, MD; Hunter Wessells, MD; Andrew P. Windsperger, MD; Lee C. Zhao, MD, MS.

The planning committee, staff, authors and editors listed below have identified financial relationships or relationships to products or devices they or their spouse/life partner have with commercial interest related to the content of this CME activity:
Allen F. Morey, MD is a consultant/advisor for AMS, and is on speakers bureau for AMS, Coloplast Group, and GlaxoSmithKline.

Samir S. Taneja, MD is on Speakers Bureau for Janssen Pharmaceuticals, Inc., and is a consultant/advisor for Elgen, GTx, Inc., Bayer HealthCare Pharmaceuticals and HealthTronics, Inc.

UNAPPROVED/OFF-LABEL USE DISCLOSURE
The EOCME requires CME faculty to disclose to the participants:
1. When products or procedures being discussed are off-label, unlabelled, experimental, and/or investigational (not US Food and Drug Administration (FDA) approved); and
2. Any limitations on the information presented, such as data that are preliminary or that represent ongoing research, interim analyses, and/or unsupported opinions. Faculty may discuss information about pharmaceutical agents that is outside of FDA-approved labelling. This information is intended solely for CME and is not intended to promote off-label use of these medications. If you have any questions, contact the medical affairs department of the manufacturer for the most recent prescribing information.

TO ENROLL
To enroll in the *Urologic Clinics of North America* Continuing Medical Education program, call customer service at 1-800-654-2452 or sign up online at http://www.theclinics.com/home/cme. The CME program is available to subscribers for an additional annual fee of $243 USD.

METHOD OF PARTICIPATION
In order to claim credit, participants must complete the following:
1. Complete enrolment as indicated above.
2. Read the activity.
3. Complete the CME Test and Evaluation. Participants must achieve a score of 70% on the test. All CME Tests and Evaluations must be completed online.

CME INQUIRIES/SPECIAL NEEDS
For all CME inquiries or special needs, please contact elsevierCME@elsevier.com.

UROLOGIC CLINICS OF NORTH AMERICA

NOW AVAILABLE FOR YOUR iPhone and iPad

Foreword

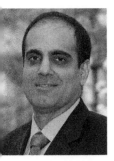

Samir S. Taneja, MD
Consulting Editor

This issue of the *Urologic Clinics* is devoted to the field of genitourinary trauma and reconstruction. While reconstructive procedures often are for the correction of anatomic abnormalities arising from iatrogenic and traumatic origin, surgeons subspecializing in trauma are uniquely experienced to provide insight into reconstructive procedures for correction of a wide multitude of etiologies. As such, I am confident the articles provided in this issue will provide a valuable resource for urologists in all types of clinical practice.

Reconstruction of the urinary tract is a mainstay of urologic practice. While we often define reconstructive surgery as a procedure specifically intended to correct a pre-existing problem, the surgical principles arising from our reconstructive procedures can and should influence the vast majority of procedures performed in urology. Reconstructive principles can be applied in oncologic procedures requiring reconstruction following extirpation, general urologic procedures, correction of congenital abnormalities, and in the management of complications arising from urologic surgery.

Similarly, the management of genitourinary trauma offers insight into the management of common challenges arising from renal surgery, lower urinary tract surgery, and secondary surgical complications. We can learn a great deal, for example, on how to manage partial nephrectomy complications through the observation of our colleagues experienced with both penetrating and blunt renal trauma. While many urologists in practice do not manage acute trauma, almost all are exposed to iatrogenic trauma arising from both urologic and nonurologic surgical procedures.

In this issue, Dr Allen Morey and Dr Steven Hudak have crafted a comprehensive look into the contemporary management of urologic trauma and the strategies for reconstruction of traumatic sequelae. I am deeply indebted to Drs Morey and Hudak for insight into the design of this issue and oversight in its creation. Each of the authors has provided a unique perspective to the principles of reconstruction as they may be applied in different regions of the urinary tract, and in both the acute and the delayed setting. I would like to thank each of the authors for these fantastic articles. I urge the readers to absorb the concepts to take back to everyday practice.

Samir S. Taneja, MD
Division of Urologic Oncology
Smilow Comprehensive Prostate Cancer Center
Department of Urology
NYU Langone Medical Center
150 East 32nd Street, Suite 200
New York, NY 10016, USA

E-mail address:
samir.taneja@nyumc.org

Urol Clin N Am 40 (2013) xi
http://dx.doi.org/10.1016/j.ucl.2013.05.002
0094-0143/13/$ – see front matter

Preface
Urologic Trauma and Reconstruction

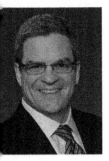 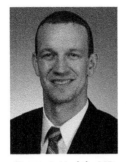

Allen F. Morey, MD   Steven J. Hudak, MD
Editors

During the last three decades, genitourinary reconstructive surgery has evolved dramatically. With increasing numbers of fellowship programs in urologic reconstruction now in existence across the country, expertise is now available in the majority of academic programs and large group practices nationwide. Graduating urology residents now enter the general urologic community with a solid foundation in genitourinary reconstructive surgery as well as minimally invasive surgical techniques. In this issue of *The Urologic Clinics*, we have attempted to present a current, state-of-the-art examination of clinically relevant challenges encountered by urologists managing acute urologic trauma or performing delayed genitourinary reconstruction.

Urologic injury often occurs in the context of severe multisystem trauma, which requires close cooperation with trauma surgeons. The urologist remains an important consultant to the trauma team, helping to ensure that the structure and function of the genitourinary system is preserved whenever possible. Immediate interventions for acute urologic injuries often require flexibility in accordance with damage control principles in critically ill patients. Minimally invasive techniques for

achieving hemostasis have become mainstream among renal trauma patients, and this version of *The Urologic Clinics* identifies important radiographic predictors of those who may benefit from urgent angiographic intervention. The role of robotic surgery, having changed the face of urologic oncology, is now increasingly employed in complex ureteral reconstruction, especially for distal strictures.

The acute management of pelvic fracture–associated urethral injuries remains an ongoing controversy. Primary endoscopic urethral realignment is presented with important recommendations for patient selection and procedural conduct. Many of these patients will ultimately require posterior urethral reconstruction, which remains the hallmark operation for reconstructive urologists, and technical considerations for optimal outcomes are reviewed.

Significant reconstructive challenges often await the urologic trauma patient who has recovered from his associated injuries. Genital injuries are rarely life-threatening, but often become the male trauma patient's chief concern once acute issues are resolved. Plastic surgical principles offer

The opinions expressed in this document are solely those of the authors and do not represent an endorsement by or the views of the United States Air Force, the United States Army, the Department of Defense or the United States Government.

Urol Clin N Am 40 (2013) xiii–xiv
http://dx.doi.org/10.1016/j.ucl.2013.05.001
0094-0143/13/$ – see front matter © 2013 Published by Elsevier Inc.

an important guide for optimal genital cosmesis and function. Similarly, complex proximal ureteral defects are often not amenable to robotic repair; classic reconstructive techniques, such as Boari flap, ileal ureter, and downward nephropexy, remain commonplace in the robotic era. Finally, although advances in prostate cancer management continue to improve outcomes and decrease morbidity, many men will ultimately encounter negative sequelae from oncologic treatment. Two separate articles in this issue of *The Urologic Clinics* are devoted to the management of 2 of the most challenging iatrogenic conditions facing urologists: radiation-induced lower genitourinary injuries and refractory postprostatectomy bladder neck contractures.

Effective rehabilitation of the urologic trauma patient remains an immensely gratifying undertaking. As the field of genitourinary reconstruction continues to evolve, we must strive to approac clinical problems in a creative, yet evidence based manner to ensure optimal outcomes.

Allen F. Morey, M
Department of Urolog
UT Southwestern Medical Cente
5323 Harry Hines Boulevar
Dallas, TX 75390-9110, US.

Steven J. Hudak, M
Department of Surgery, Urology Sectio
San Antonio Military Medical Cente
3851 Roger Brooke Driv
Fort Sam Houston, TX 78234, US.

E-mail addresse:
allen.morey@utsouthwestern.edu (A.F. Morey
steven.j.hudak2.mil@mail.mil (S.J. Huda

Current Epidemiology of Genitourinary Trauma

James B. McGeady, MD, Benjamin N. Breyer, MD, MAS*

KEYWORDS

• Urologic • Trauma • Epidemiology • Kidney • Ureter • Bladder • Urethra • Genitalia

KEY POINTS

- With 10% of the 2.8 million trauma patients hospitalized yearly in the United States sustaining genitourinary injuries, an understanding of the epidemiology of genitourinary organ injury facilitates prompt diagnosis and appropriate treatment of these injuries.
- The use of national data sets to conduct large population-based studies has increased our understanding of the epidemiology of genitourinary trauma.
- Most renal, bladder, and posterior urethral trauma is from blunt mechanisms, most commonly motor vehicle collisions.
- Most ureteral and anterior urethral injuries are iatrogenic.
- Research and development of safer vehicles along with public efforts and policy to create safer roadways and regulate hazardous driving activities continues to decrease morbidity and mortality from motor vehicle collisions.

INTRODUCTION

The importance of recognizing and appropriately managing urogenital injuries has been appreciated for centuries. Timely identification and management of these injuries is often organ saving, and at times, life saving.

Worldwide, trauma is currently the sixth leading cause of death, accounting for 10% of mortalities.[1] In the United States, more than 2.8 million people are hospitalized as a result of trauma yearly, with estimated costs of $406 billion annually in medical expenditures and lost productivity.[2] Trauma has a predilection for young adults and results in the loss of more productive work years than cancer and heart disease combined.[3] The urogenital system has consistently been shown to be involved in 10% of patients presenting after trauma and is therefore a significant factor in trauma-induced morbidity and mortality.[4]

Most trauma data from the 20th century were reported from single-institution data sets. With the expansion of electronic medical records and national trauma networks, national data sets have become a more accessible and significant source of information.

The National Electronic Injury Surveillance System (NEISS), originally created in 1970 by the US Consumer Product Safety Commission, is one example of these national data sets. It has been used primarily to evaluate the magnitude of injury associated with consumer products, but because it provides a national probability estimate of all injury-related US emergency department presentations, it has proved to be a useful tool for evaluating many facets of trauma epidemiology.

More recently, the National Trauma Data Bank (NTDB), created in 1989, has continued to grow exponentially and currently contains more than 5 million records, making it by far the largest national data set available. It has been increasingly analyzed over the last 2 decades, resulting in significant contributions to the medical literature

Department of Urology, University of California, 400 Parnassus Avenue, Suite A-610, San Francisco, CA 94143, USA
* Corresponding author.
E-mail address: bbreyer@urology.ucsf.edu

Urol Clin N Am 40 (2013) 323–334
http://dx.doi.org/10.1016/j.ucl.2013.04.001
0094-0143/13/$ – see front matter © 2013 Elsevier Inc. All rights reserved.

and increased understanding of trauma incidence, mechanism, and outcomes.[5]

The Crash Research and Engineering (CIREN) database, which is a multicenter research network developed by the National Highway Traffic Safety Administration, provides detailed crash site analysis and specific occupant injury data to help researchers better understand the mechanisms of injury in motor vehicle collisions (MVC).

Although far from comprehensive, these are several important examples of the major data sets relating to trauma. In the future, as the evaluation and sharing of data become easier and faster, the continued development of more inclusive and refined data sets will enable researchers to probe further into the epidemiology and, hopefully, prevention of trauma.

ORGANS
Kidney

Prevalence/incidence
Renal injury has historically been reported in 1.2% to 3.3% of trauma patients depending on the data

Europe.[10] Penetrating injuries are more prevalent in undeveloped countries and areas with civil unrest. A retrospective, 4-year single-institution study from a hospital serving 13 smaller cities throughout southeastern Turkey, a region with elevated sociopolitical tensions and a gun in every residence for self-defense and hunting reported 59% (42/71) of renal injuries were secondary to gunshot wounds (GSW).[11] Similarly 75% (130/174) of renal injuries reported by one hospital in Durban, South Africa were from a penetrating source, with 50% (87/174) caused by GSW.[12] Although penetrating renal injury which is responsible for 16% of renal injuries per review of the NTDB, is much less common than blunt renal trauma, the incidence of civilian GSW is reportedly increasing in the United States, Africa, and some European countries.[9,13] Of traumatized patients in the United States, the proportion with renal injury was highest in those sustaining injuries from firearms (3.5%), MVC (2.2%), bicycle accidents (1.9%), pedestrian accidents (1.5%), stab wounds (0.8%), and falls (0.5%).[9]

The epidemiology of renal trauma—Summary of multiple series

	Rate of Renal Injury (%)	Number	Blunt (%)	Penetrating (%)	Minor Injuries (%)	Major Injuries (%)[a]	Renal Exploration (%)	Nephrectomy (%)
Seattle[7]	2.8	154	93.5	6.5	92	8	N/A	3.8
Toronto[14]	3.25	132	95.4	4.6	72	28	7.4	3.2
San Francisco[6]	N/A	2254	89.8	10.2	91.1	8.9	7.4	0.8
British Columbia[8]	1.4	227	93.4	6.6	81.7	18.3	7.1	N/A
NTDB[9]	1.2	6231	81.6	16.0	82.5	17.5	13	7

[a] Major injury defined as AAST grades 2 to 5 or ICD-9 code for laceration, parenchymal disruption, or vascular injury.
Data from Wessells H, Suh D, Porter JR, et al. Renal injury and operative management in the United States: results of a population-based study. J Trauma 2003;54(3):423–30.

set.[6–8] A recent population-based study using the NTDB and consisting of 6231 renal injuries found an incidence of 4.9 per 100,000 population.[9] Like other trauma, renal injuries are also associated with youth and male gender. Renal injuries occurred in patients less than 44 years of age 70% to 80% of the time and almost 75% of these were male.[9]

Mechanism
In the United States, 82% to 95% of renal injuries are secondary to blunt trauma,[9] slightly less than the 93% observed in Canada[8] and 97% in

Motor vehicle collisions
MVC account for approximately 70% of blunt renal injuries, with 50.9% involving 2 vehicles, 21.1% involving a solitary vehicle, and 11.1% involving vehicle versus pedestrian.[15,16] According to the World Health Organization, approximately 1.3 million people die yearly from road traffic accidents, and another 20 to 50 million suffer nonfatal injuries.[17] Ongoing research into preventative measures to lessen solid organ injury has provided insight into the mechanism of renal injury in various MVC scenarios, as well as the effects of multiple automobile safety features.

ne of these studies, a recent review of the JREN database, demonstrated a 45.3% and 2.8% reduction in renal injury during collisions ith frontal and side airbags, respectively.[18] In a eparate analysis of the same data set, seat belts, hich unquestionably decrease overall morbidity nd mortality in accidents, have been shown to ccount for 90% of renal injuries in frontal colliions.[19] Side-door panel/armrest direct impact is ne source of renal injury in most side-impact colsions, as is the steering wheel and instrument anel for unrestrained drivers in head-on collions. Interestingly, although not statistically sigificant, renal injury was more likely on the right ide for restrained drivers and left for restrained assengers, possibly due to the lower/mid bdominal location of the shoulder restraint on ne medial side.[19]

icycles

Vith 57 million, or 27% of the US population over ne age of 16, riding bicycles on a daily basis, inries sustained from bicycle-related accidents ontribute significantly to the trauma population. ccording to a review of mode-by-mode fatality nd travel statistics report from the US Department of Transportation by Pucher and Dijkstra, icycling is considered 12 times more likely to esult in mortality than riding in a car per kilometer traveled, and results in greater than 600 eaths annually.[20,21] A review of the 16,585 icycle-related trauma cases in the NTDB noted hat genitourinary (GU) trauma occurred in 2% f bicycle accidents (358 patients).[20] Renal rauma was the most common type of GU injury n this subset (75%–80% of GU injuries), with ladder and urethral injuries a distant secnd.[16,20,22] A review of the NEISS database estinated that 43,542 (95% confidence interval [CI] 6,447–50,363), or 9%, of all GU injuries presentng to US emergency departments from 2002 to 010 had a bicycle-related injury.[23] Of these njuries, 31% (12,707 [95% CI 9585–15,830]) nvolved the testicles or scrotum, with renal injury epresenting only 5% (2158 [95% CI 1360–2956]) f GU injuries presenting to the emergency oom.[23] This discrepancy is likely due to the ifferent patient populations represented by the ITDB and NEISS. Patients in the NTDB have njuries significant enough to require hospital dmission and therefore are more likely to have renal injury. The NEISS database, on the other and, includes all emergency department preentations, most of which are treated in an mbulatory setting, and not surprisingly consist f a significantly higher number of scrotal njuries.[23]

Pediatrics

Because of children's weaker abdominal muscles, less ossified and protective rib cage, paucity of perirenal fat, intra-abdominal renal location, and relatively larger kidney-to-body size ratio, they have an increased risk of blunt renal injury.[24] Approximately 10% of children presenting with blunt abdominal trauma have a renal injury.[25] According to a recent review of the NEISS database, there were approximately 8249 pediatric renal injuries that presented to emergency rooms in the United States between 2002 and 2010. Although renal injuries accounted for only 3.5% of all pediatric GU injuries, it was responsible for 25.7% of hospital admissions in this cohort.[26]

All-terrain vehicles (ATVs)

The use of ATVs in both the general and the pediatric populations has continued to increase over the last 20 years. Despite government legislation, multiple public awareness campaigns, improved safety labeling, and age-appropriate recommendations from numerous organizations, ATVs are responsible for an increasing number of pediatric injuries and deaths each year. An estimated 28,300 children under the age of 16 years of age presented to the emergency department in 2010 with ATV-related injuries and there have been 2775 reported deaths since 1982.[27] Several recent single-institutional retrospective studies evaluated the risk of GU injury in this subset of patients. Approximately 3% to 3.7% of ATV-related pediatric admissions sustained GU trauma, which was overwhelmingly renal in nature (22/23 patients, 96%).[28,29] In contrast to a previous publication whereby a rollover injury or a blow to the abdomen from the handlebars was the source of renal injury, ejection was identified as the predominant mechanism of ATV-related pediatric injury in these more recent cohorts.[29,30]

Sports and solitary kidneys

There has been a significant amount of ambiguity regarding the appropriate recommendations for children with solitary kidneys who wish to participate in contact sports. According to 182 responses to a survey sent to 231 active members of the American Academy of Pediatrics in 2002, 68% of these practitioners reported that they recommend patients with a solitary kidney avoid contact sports.[31]

Since 1994, the American Academy of Pediatrics has recommended a "qualified yes" pending assessment for children with solitary kidneys wishing to participate in contact sports.[32] In 2012 Grinsell and colleagues[33] used the data collected for the National Athletic Trainers' Association

Injury Surveillance Study, an observational cohort study collected during the 1995 to 1997 academic years, to evaluate the risk of renal injury in contact/collision sports. From 1995 to 1997, more than 4.4 million athlete-exposures, defined as 1 athlete participating in 1 game or practice, were evaluated and 23,666 physical injuries were reported. Eighteen minor kidney injuries, 3 lacerations, and 15 contusions were observed. None of these injuries required surgical management or resulted in known loss of renal function. For boys, football had the highest rate of renal injury (9.2 injuries/million athlete-exposures). Girls had the highest risk of sustaining a renal injury while playing soccer (5.9 injuries/million athlete-exposures). Overall, the risk of renal injury was significantly less than rates of traumatic brain/head/neck/spine injuries and it was concluded that patients with solitary kidneys should be allowed to participate in contact sports.[33]

Ureter

Prevalence/incidence

Ureteral trauma is rare. Almost 25 years ago a large single-institution retrospective study reported ureteral injury in 1% of all urologic trauma.[34] More recently, a retrospective analysis of the 22,706 GU injuries in the NTDB from 2002 to 2006 found ureteral trauma responsible for 2.5% of GU trauma (582 patients total).[35] This significantly increased incidence is attributed to improved evacuation, stabilization, and evaluation methods of trauma patients resulting in increased survival of severely injured patients with improved initial detection of ureteral injuries.[35]

A recent literature review on ureteral trauma published by Pereira and colleagues[36] identified 77 articles with level 3 to 4 evidence. Consistent with the observation that most trauma occurs in young men, the reviewers noted that an average of 83.4% of patients with ureteral trauma were men, on average 23.2 years of age. This male predominance, which is even higher than for overall trauma, may be representative of the strong association of ureteral injuries with penetrating trauma (61%–62%).[35]

Mechanism/location

A review of the NTDB from 2002 to 2006 noted that penetrating ureteral injuries occur in a significantly younger population than blunt injuries, 27 versus 37 years of age, respectively (P<.001), and are more likely to occur in men than blunt injuries (91% vs 73%).[35] Interestingly, this review also demonstrated a much higher overall percentage of ureteral injuries from blunt mechanisms than previously published (38% vs 3%).[37] Most

penetrating ureteral injuries (88%) were secondary to GSW, whereas most blunt injuries were associated with MVC (50%). A recent 25-year review of ureteral trauma at the San Francisco General Hospital described the location of 38 ureteral injuries as 70% upper, 8% mid, and 22% distal.[36,3] Most of the upper ureteral injuries were described as short segment losses amenable to repair with a tension-free anastomosis after initial debridement.[38]

Mechanisms of ureteral injury per NTDB review		
	N = 528	Total Cases (%)
Blunt trauma	24	38
MVC	110	19
Pedestrian	25	4
Motorcyclist	18	3
High fall	15	3
Low fall	8	1
Cyclist	3	<1
Other	45	8
Penetrating trauma	358	62
Gunshot wound	316	54
Stab	29	5
Other	13	2

Data from Siram SM, Gerald SZ, Greene WR, et al. Ureteral trauma: patterns and mechanisms of injury of an uncommon condition. Am J Surg 2010;199(4):566–70.

Concurrent injuries

Associated injuries are present in 90.4% of trauma patients with ureteral injury.[36] This association represents the ureter's approximation to many abdominal and retroperitoneal organs as well as the severity, and often penetrating nature, of the insult needed to cause a ureteral injury.[39] Siram and colleagues[35] found the colon/appendix (51%) and small intestine (49%) to be the most commonly associated injuries, which is consistent with findings of previous single-institution studies.[36] Surprisingly though, their data showed a much greater incidence of vessel injury with penetrating trauma than previously described by Perez-Brayfield and colleagues[40] (38% vs 13%).[35] Congruent with previous single-institution series, Siram and colleagues[35] also found a higher incidence of arterial injuries with blunt rather than penetrating trauma (9% vs 5% respectively). The converse is true for penetrating trauma whereby venous injuries occurred 27% of the time and arterial injuries were seen in 16%. The iliac vessels lie just posterior to the ureters as they enter the bony pelvis and are especially susceptible to injury at this location, which explains how together they are injured in 28% of penetrating trauma. Not surprisingly, patients with blunt trauma and ureteral injuries are much more likely to have associated orthopedic injuries than penetrating cases (20% vs 1%).[35]

Iatrogenic ureteral injury

According to the Consensus on GU Trauma statement on diagnosis and management of ureteric injury by Brandes and colleagues[41] and McAninch, gyenocologic surgery accounts for greater than half of all iatrogenic ureteric injuries. A systematic review of benign gynecologic surgery estimated that ureteral injury ranged from 0.2 to 7.3 per 1000 surgeries.[42] Although ureteral injury typically occurs during gynecologic, urologic, urogynecologic, and other pelvic surgeries, it has been reported with something as simple as a Foley catheter placement.[41,43,44]

The pelvic ureter is involved in 80% of iatrogenic ureteral injuries, making it by far the most commonly involved segment.[45] The most common types of ureteral injury, in decreasing order of frequency, are ligation, kinking by suture, transection/avulsion, partial transection, crush, and devascularization with delayed necrosis/stricture.[41] Prior studies have identified resection of large pelvic masses, malignant neoplasms, inflammatory disease, laparoscopy, and prior operation or radiation therapy as risk factors for iatrogenic ureteral injury.[46,47] These injuries generally occur in the distal one-third of the ureter and are not prevented by placement of preoperative stents, although they do assist with intraoperative recognition when they occur.

8565 patients with documented bladder injury. Of the subjects, 75% were men and 57% were under 40 years (mean 38.9 years). A retrospective single-institution study previously found 1.6% of blunt trauma patients had a bladder injury.[51] In 2009 Bjurlin and colleagues[52] reviewed the 1,466,887 patient records in the NTDB between 2001 and 2005 and found that 3.6% of patients presenting with a pelvic fracture had a concomitant bladder injury. Although men are more likely to engage in risky activities that result in a pelvic fracture, they noted that men and women presenting with pelvic fracture had a similar incidence of isolated bladder ruptures (3.41% vs 3.37%, $P = .848$).[52] Several large literature reviews have found that extraperitoneal bladder ruptures make up most injuries (55%–78%), with the rest consisting of intraperitoneal (17%–39%) and combined intraperitoneal and extraperitoneal (5%–8%) ruptures.[53,54]

Blunt bladder trauma

Blunt trauma accounts for most bladder ruptures (51%–86%).[51,55,56] The 2004 "Consensus Statement on Bladder Injuries" noted that a pelvic fracture increased the likelihood of bladder rupture from 1.6% to 5.7%, which is slightly more than the 3.6% described in the NTDB review.[53] A 20-year prospectively maintained database recently reported that MVCs are the most common cause of blunt bladder rupture (50.5%) followed by pedestrians versus automobile (29.1%), and falling from a great height (14.5%).[55] Pelvic fractures are present 70% (35%–90%) of the time there is a bladder rupture, which demonstrates the strong association between these conditions.[50,57] Specific pelvic injuries, notably diastasis

Incidence of specific organ injury in patients with GU trauma						
	NEISS[48]	Scotland[49]	GSW[13]	MVC[16]	Bicycles[20,23]	Motorcycles[16]
Kidney	7.7%	67%	54%	65%	5%–75%	28%
Ureter	N/A	3%	3.8%	0	N/A	0
Bladder	N/A	18%	18.7%	16%	13%	5%
Urethra	N/A	16%	2.9%	2%	9%	3%[a]
External genitalia	74.3%	20%	29.4%	17%	13%–31%	64%

[a] Multiple GU organs may be injured in an individual trauma patient.

Bladder

Prevalence/incidence

Due to its protected location within the bony pelvis, bladder injuries are not as common as their renal counterpart, but still occur with both blunt and penetrating trauma. Deibert and Spencer[50] reviewed the NTDB from 2002 to 2006 and identified

of the symphysis pubis or sacroiliac joints and displaced fractures of the obturator ring or pubic rami, have been shown to be associated with bladder rupture.[58] Most bladder ruptures without an associated pelvic fracture occur after a hard blow to the abdomen in a person with a distended bladder, often resulting in an intraperitoneal blowout injury of the bladder dome. The associated mortality rate of 10% to 22% for patients with a bladder rupture demonstrates the high-energy and multisystem trauma that is usually involved.[56]

Penetrating bladder trauma

The percentage of bladder injuries caused by a penetrating mechanism range from 14% to 49% in several large single series and NTDB reviews, with GSW comprising the vast majority (88%, 316/358 patients with penetrating injury).[50,55] Per a large literature review, penetrating bladder injury is reported in 3.6% of abdominal GSW, 13% of penetrating injuries to the rectum, and 20% of penetrating injuries to the buttock.[53]

Iatrogenic bladder injury

Iatrogenic bladder injury is not uncommon. It is the most frequently injured organ during obstetric and gynecologic procedures, with a rising incidence paralleling the rise in complexity of the surgery (1.8–13.8 per 1000 surgeries).[44,59] Other reported miscellaneous causes for bladder injury reported in literature include trocar placement in the emergency setting for diagnostic laparoscopy,[60] during orthopedic treatment of pelvic fractures with external fixators,[61] and placement of an intrauterine device.[62]

Operative risk of iatrogenic bladder injury	
Injury Type	Frequency per 1000 Procedures
Open radical hysterectomy	14
Laparoscopic-assisted vaginal hysterectomy	13.8
Laparoscopic hysterectomy	10
Vaginal hysterectomy	9
Cesarean section	1.8
Laparoscopic herniorrhaphy	1.6
Mid urethral sling	0.4
Vaginal delivery	0.1

Data from Gomez RG, Ceballos L, Coburn M, et al. Consensus statement on bladder injuries. BJU Int 2004;94(1):27–32.

Bladder neck injury

Bladder neck injuries secondary to blunt trauma in prepubescent boys are well described in the urologic literature. The increased prevalence in this age group over adults is thought to be secondary to their undeveloped prostate. Consequently, there is minimal literature beyond case reports describing pelvic fracture–related injuries of the bladder neck and prostate until Mundy and Andrich recently reported on 15 patients where they described the mechanism of bladder neck involvement as an extension of a primary injury to the prostate and prostatic urethra.[63]

Urethra

Prevalence/incidence

Urethral injuries are rare in the trauma population, accounting for approximately 4% of GU trauma per several series, but have the propensity to incur substantial long-term morbidity including intractable stricture disease, incontinence, impotence, and infertility.[49,64] When the urethra is injured 65% are complete disruptions with the remaining 35% resulting in partial tears.[65] Men are approximately 5 times more likely to have a urethral injury than women, which is attributed to the longer length and reduced mobility of the male urethra.[66,67]

Posterior urethral injuries

Posterior urethral injuries associated with pelvic fractures are the most common noniatrogenic urethral injury in industrialized societies and are approximately 4 times more common than anterior urethral injuries.[68] Depending on the magnitude of trauma, the posterior urethra is initially stretched and then partially or completely disrupted at the bulbomembranous junction.[69] Continued research into the mechanisms of posterior urethral injury with pelvic fractures as well as the inherent risks/associations of specific fracture types has further advanced the understanding of these injuries. A prospective study including more than 200 men with pelvic fractures demonstrated that combined straddle fracture and diastasis of the sacroiliac joint confer a 24 times higher risk of urethral injury. Straddle fracture alone has 3.85 times the risk and Malgaigne fracture increases the risk by a factor of 3.4.[70] In a retrospective, nested case-control study of 119 male patients with pelvic fracture and urethral injury, Basta and colleagues[71] found that 92% of the subjects had specific inferomedial pubic bone fractures or pubic symphysis diastasis, with 88% of these being displaced more than 1 cm. Recently, computer-generated models of the pelvis and urethra have allowed a greater understanding of the mechanisms of urethral stretching followed by disruption at the bulbo-membranous junction.[72–74]

Anterior urethral injuries

Blunt injury to the anterior urethra occurs approximately one-quarter as often as posterior injury and is generally a "straddle-type" injury of the bulbar urethra. This type of injury results from

irect trauma to the urethra itself and often results
a a partial disruption or, quite frequently, is not
nitially identified and presents later as a stric-
ure.[54] Slightly less commonly, the anterior urethra
s injured during a fracture of the penis. The
ncidence of concomitant urethral injury varies
eographically, but ranges from 0% to 3% in
sia and the Middle East to 20% to 38% in the
Inited States and Europe.[75,76] Urethral injuries
lso occur more commonly with bilateral caver-
osal tears.[77]

Penetrating injuries to the anterior urethra are
sually secondary to GSW and involve the bulbar
nd pendulous segments equally.[78] The urethra
vas injured in 2.9% of civilian GSW involving the
SU system in a retrospective review of 309 pa-
ents sustaining GSW in the Henry Ford Medical
Center Trauma Registry. Frequently there are
oncomitant lower extremity and pelvic injuries in
hese patients (44% and 33%, respectively).[13]

atrogenic urethral injury

Perhaps the most common cause of anterior ure-
hral injury is iatrogenic from Foley catheter place-
nent. Although it is difficult to identify the exact
umber of Foley catheters placed, 24 million are
old to hospitals within the United States annu-
lly.[79] A year-long, prospective, single-institution
tudy at University California, San Diego found
atheter-related injuries to occur in approximately
.2 per 1000 patients, but after implementing

Scrotal and testicular trauma

Although exposed and dependent in nature, the
mobility of the scrotum often prevents it and its
contents from severe injury. Still, traumatic injury
to the external genitalia, including the penis, is
seen in 27.8% to 68.1% of all trauma patients
with injury to the GU tract according to multiple
published series.[81,82] Blunt trauma accounts for
up to 85% of scrotal and testicular injuries, most
of which are sustained during athletic activity.[83]
Scrotal trauma can result in a spectrum of findings
ranging from local hematoma to ruptured or dislo-
cated testicles.[84]

Penetrating scrotal trauma, albeit less common,
is generally more severe and usually requires surgical exploration. Up to 40% to 60% of penetrating
GU injuries involve the external genitalia. In a
30-year single-institution retrospective review of
110 patients with penetrating external genital injuries, Phonsombat and colleagues[85] found that
gunshots account for 55% of penetrating scrotal
trauma, with stab wounds/lacerations (42%), and
bites (3%) accounting for the rest. Orchiectomy
rates range from 25% to 65% depending on the
study, with a higher prevalence in lacerations
than GSW, likely due to the high propensity of
self-inflicted orchiectomies, which are less often
salvageable.[81]

Review of published series on GSW trauma to scrotum

Institution	No. of Patients	No. of Injured Testicles (%)	No. of Nonoperative Management (%)	No. of Orchiectomies (%)
Temple Univ.[81]	97	50 (54.9)	6 (6.2)	24 (48)
UMDNJ[86]	62	33 (61.1)	8 (12.9)	20 (60.6)
UCSF[85]	40	24 (60)	0 (0)	6 (25)
LSU[87]	27	23 (85.2)	0 (0)	15 (65.2)
UCLA-Harbor[88]	19	4 (66.7)	13 (68.4)	2 (50.0)
Wash. Univ.[89]	17	17 (100)	0 (0)	6 (35.3)

ursing education programs on Foley catheter
lacement, they showed a decrease in incidence
o less than 1 per 1000 patients, illustrating the
value of these preventative measures.[80]

xternal genitalia

Due to the external location of the male genitalia,
hey are relatively exposed and vulnerable to
rauma. Although not generally life threatening,
genital injury is relatively common. Prompt
attention is warranted to limit long-term sexual,
reproductive, physiologic, and psychological
damage.

Penile trauma

Penile trauma is less common than scrotal/testic-
ular trauma, but still comprises 10% to 16% of
GU injuries per several single-institution series.[90]
In one large civilian study, penetrating penile
trauma accounted for 33% of all penetrating genital trauma (scrotum = 48%).[85] Associated urethral
injury ranges from 4% to 24% depending on the
study and mechanism. Stab wounds/lacerations
seem to have a higher likelihood of involving the
urethra than GSW.[13,85]

Penile fracture is an uncommon and likely underreported injury, accounting for 1 in every 175,000 emergency room visits.[91] Still, according to the National Inpatient Sample, a nationally representative weighted sample of hospital admission data, there were 1043 men admitted to US hospitals for penile fracture in 2006 to 2007.[92] Of the 1331 cases of penile fracture reported in the literature between 1935 and 2001, over half were from the Mediterranean region.[93] Mechanism of injury varies geographically. The practice of "taghaandan," where the erect penis is forcibly pushed down to achieve detumescence, is the most common cause in the Mediterranean region.[94] In the United States and Europe, most fractures occur after the penis slips out of the vagina during intercourse and thrusts against the perineum or pubic symphysis.[95] A retrospective chart review of 16 patients presenting to the University of Maryland with penile fracture found that intercourse in stressful situations, specifically out-of-the-ordinary locations (68.7%) and extramarital affairs (43.8%), seems to be a common theme in these patients.[96]

Military trauma

The ever-changing landscape of warfare and the institution of Kevlar body armor have likely affected the mechanism and distribution of GU injury seen in modern combat. Historically, GU injury constituted a small portion of battlefield injuries, ranging from 0.7% to 8%, with renal injury noted in up to 40%.[97–99] Most of these wounds resulted from bullet injury. Now, projectile fragments from mortar shells, aerial bombs, rockets, and improvised explosive devices account for most modern battlefield urologic injuries.[97]

Recent reports from overseas contingency operations the US Military is currently engaged in have reported similar findings with GU involvement in 2.8% to 5% of injuries.[98,100] The largest cohort, consisting of 16,323 trauma admissions, reported 887 GU injuries with involvement of the scrotum in 257 (29%), kidney in 203 (22.9%), bladder in 189 (21.3%), penis in 126 (14.2%), testicle in 81 (9.1%), ureter in 24 (2.7%), and urethra in 7 (0.8%).[100] Explosive devices were responsible for 50% to 65% of the injuries; individual firearms caused 15% to 37%, and the remaining 11% to 13% were due to blunt injury, primarily MVC.[98,100]

The shift in primary mechanism of injury, from penetrating missile to explosive fragments, and the increased use of body armor have changed the spectrum of injuries seen on the battlefield. The higher rate of genital injury (68%) seen in soldiers in recent conflicts is likely because of explosions.[100,101] The decreased renal and ureteral injuries are likely a result of protective body armor.[97,98,102]

RESEARCH FUTURE DIRECTIONS

At the time of establishment of the Centers for Disease Control and Prevention injury center in 1987, only 5 centers, including Harvard University, Johns Hopkins University, University of North Carolina, University of Washington, and Wayne State University, were funded. Today the injury center funds 11 programs, and vast improvements continue to be noted in multiple injury areas. For example, in 2010, 32,885 people died in motor vehicle traffic crashes in the United States—the lowest number of fatalities since 1949 and 2.9% decline from 2009 (33,883 fatalities).[103]

Continued research and development of safer vehicles along with public efforts and policy to create safer roadways and regulate hazardous driving activities will likely further promote this trend.

The application of computer-generated models based off of human imaging to traffic accident modeling has given us insight into the understanding of the mechanics of posterior urethral injury.[73,104]

On a different note, the recognition of violence as a public health problem has resulted in multiple evidence-based strategies and programs to reduce violence, especially in youths, and highlighted the cost-effectiveness of monetary allocations aimed at prevention instead of incarceration.[105]

As we continue into the 21st century armed with more efficient diagnostic machinery, communication and data storage technology, and tools that enable us to provide more efficient and higher quality patient care, we must continue to advance our understanding of the epidemiology of trauma to better prevent it, and more effectively treat it when it does occur.

REFERENCES

1. Smith J, Greaves I, Porter K. Major trauma. 1 publ edition. Oxford (United Kingdom): Oxford University Press; 2010. p. 1.
2. Haider AH, Saleem T, Leow JJ, et al. Influence of the National Trauma Data Bank on the study of trauma outcomes: is it time to set research best practices to further enhance its impact? J Am Coll Surg 2012;214(5):756–68.
3. Comittee on Injury Prevention and Treatment, Institute of Medicine. Reducing the burden of injury: advancing prevention and treatment. Washington, DC: National Academy Press; 1999.

4. Shewakramani S, Reed KC. Genitourinary trauma. Emerg Med Clin North Am 2011;29(3):501–18.

5. Bank, NTD. National Trauma Data Standard Data Dictionary: 2011 Admissions. Available at: http://www.ntdsdictionary.org/dataElements/documents/NTDS2011_Final3.pdf. Accessed December 4, 2012.

6. Miller KS, McAninch JW. Radiographic assessment of renal trauma: our 15-year experience. J Urol 1995;154(2 Pt 1):352–5.

7. Krieger JN, Algood CB, Mason JT, et al. Urological trauma in the Pacific Northwest: etiology, distribution, management and outcome. J Urol 1984; 132(1):70–3.

8. Baverstock R, Simons R, McLoughlin M. Severe blunt renal trauma: a 7-year retrospective review from a provincial trauma centre. Can J Urol 2001; 8(5):1372–6.

9. Wessells H, Suh D, Porter JR, et al. Renal injury and operative management in the United States: results of a population-based study. J Trauma 2003;54(3):423–30.

10. Dobrowolski Z, Kusionowicz J, Drewniak T, et al. Renal and ureteric trauma: diagnosis and management in Poland. BJU Int 2002;89(7):748–51.

11. Ersay A, Akgun Y. Experience with renal gunshot injuries in a rural setting. Urology 1999;54(6):972–5.

12. Madiba TE, Haffejee AA, John J. Renal trauma secondary to stab, blunt and firearm injuries–a 5-year study. S Afr J Surg 2002;40(1):5–9 [discussion: 9–10].

13. Najibi S, Tannast M, Latini JM. Civilian gunshot wounds to the genitourinary tract: incidence, anatomic distribution, associated injuries, and outcomes. Urology 2010;76(4):977–81 [discussion: 981].

14. Herschorn S, Radomski SB, Shoskes DA, et al. Evaluation and treatment of blunt renal trauma. J Urol 1991;146(2):274–6 [discussion: 276–7].

15. Bank, NTD. National Trauma Data Bank 2012 Annual Report. 2012. Available at: http://www.facs.org/trauma/ntdb/pdf/ntdb-annual-report-2012.pdf. Accessed December 8, 2012.

16. Paparel P, N'Diaye A, Laumon B, et al. The epidemiology of trauma of the genitourinary system after traffic accidents: analysis of a register of over 43,000 victims. BJU Int 2006;97(2):338–41.

17. Organization, WH. Road traffic injuries: fact sheet. Available at: http://www.who.int/mediacentre/factsheets/fs358/en/index.html. Accessed December 9, 2012.

18. Smith TG 3rd, Wessells HB, Mack CD, et al. Examination of the impact of airbags on renal injury using a national database. J Am Coll Surg 2010; 211(3):355–60.

19. Kuan JK, Kaufman R, Wright JL, et al. Renal injury mechanisms of motor vehicle collisions: analysis of the crash injury research and engineering network data set. J Urol 2007;178(3 Pt 1):935–40 [discussion: 940].

20. Bjurlin MA, Zhao LC, Goble SM, et al. Bicycle-related genitourinary injuries. Urology 2011;78(5):1187–90.

21. Pucher J, Dijkstra L. Promoting safe walking and cycling to improve public health: lessons from The Netherlands and Germany. Am J Public Health 2003;93(9):1509–16.

22. Lustenberger T, Inaba K, Talving P, et al. Bicyclists injured by automobiles: relationship of age to injury type and severity–a national trauma databank analysis. J Trauma 2010;69(5):1120–5.

23. Bagga HS, Breyer BN. Re: Bjurlin et al. Bicycle-related genitourinary injuries (Urology. 2011;78(5):1187-1190). Urology 2012;79(6):1415 [author reply: 1415–6].

24. Brown SL, Elder JS, Spirnak JP. Are pediatric patients more susceptible to major renal injury from blunt trauma? A comparative study. J Urol 1998; 160(1):138–40.

25. McAninch JW, Carroll PR, Klosterman PW, et al. Renal reconstruction after injury. J Urol 1991; 145(5):932–7.

26. Tasian GE, Bagga HS, Fisher PB, et al. Pediatric genitourinary injuries in the United States from 2002 to 2010. J Urol 2013;189(1):288–94.

27. Garland S. 2010 annual report of ATV-related deaths and injuries. Consumer Product Safety Commission; 2011. Available at: www.cpsc.gov/library/foia/foia12/os/atv2010.pdf. Accessed December 13, 2012.

28. Kluemper C, Rogers A, Fallat M, et al. Genitourinary injuries in pediatric all-terrain vehicle trauma–a mechanistic relationship? Urology 2010; 75(5):1162–4.

29. Hale N, Brown A. Mechanistic relationship of all-terrain vehicles and pediatric renal trauma. Urology 2013;81(1):160–2.

30. Helmkamp JC. Adolescent all-terrain vehicle deaths in West Virginia, 1990-1998. W V Med J 2000;96(1):361–3.

31. Sharp DS, Ross JH, Kay R. Attitudes of pediatric urologists regarding sports participation by children with a solitary kidney. J Urol 2002; 168(4 Pt 2):1811–4 [discussion: 1815].

32. Medical conditions affecting sports participation. American Academy of Pediatrics Committee on Sports Medicine and Fitness. Pediatrics 1994; 94(5):757–60.

33. Grinsell MM, Butz K, Gurka MJ, et al. Sport-related kidney injury among high school athletes. Pediatrics 2012;130(1):e40–5.

34. Presti JC Jr, Carroll PR, McAninch JW. Ureteral and renal pelvic injuries from external trauma: diagnosis and management. J Trauma 1989;29(3):370–4.

35. Siram SM, Gerald SZ, Greene WR, et al. Ureteral trauma: patterns and mechanisms of injury of an uncommon condition. Am J Surg 2010;199(4):566–70.

36. Pereira BM, Ogilvie MP, Gomez-Rodriguez JC, et al. A review of ureteral injuries after external trauma. Scand J Trauma Resusc Emerg Med 2010;18:6.

37. Best CD, Petrone P, Buscarini M, et al. Traumatic ureteral injuries: a single institution experience validating the American Association for the Surgery of Trauma-Organ Injury Scale grading scale. J Urol 2005;173(4):1202–5.

38. Elliott SP, McAninch JW. Ureteral injuries from external violence: the 25-year experience at San Francisco General Hospital. J Urol 2003; 170(4 Pt 1):1213–6.

39. Bent C, Iyngkaran T, Power N, et al. Urological injuries following trauma. Clin Radiol 2008;63(12): 1361–71.

40. Perez-Brayfield MR, Keane TE, Krishnan A, et al. Gunshot wounds to the ureter: a 40-year experience at Grady Memorial Hospital. J Urol 2001; 166(1):119–21.

41. Brandes S, Coburn M, Armenakas N, et al. Diagnosis and management of ureteric injury: an evidence-based analysis. BJU Int 2004;94(3):277–89.

42. Gilmour DT, Das S, Flowerdew G. Rates of urinary tract injury from gynecologic surgery and the role of intraoperative cystoscopy. Obstet Gynecol 2006;107(6):1366–72.

43. Hale N, Baugh D, Womack G. Mid-ureteral rupture: a rare complication of urethral catheterization. Urology 2012;80(5):e65–6.

44. Frankman EA, Wang L, Bunker CH, et al. Lower urinary tract injury in women in the United States, 1979-2006. Am J Obstet Gynecol 2010;202(5): 495.e1–5.

45. Klap J, Phe V, Chartier-Kastler E, et al. Aetiology and management of iatrogenic injury of the ureter: a review. Prog Urol 2012;22(15):913–9 [in French].

46. Palaniappa NC, Telem DA, Ranasinghe NE, et al. Incidence of iatrogenic ureteral injury after laparoscopic colectomy. Arch Surg 2012;147(3):267–71.

47. Parpala-Sparman T, Paananen I, Santala M, et al. Increasing numbers of ureteric injuries after the introduction of laparoscopic surgery. Scand J Urol Nephrol 2008;42(5):422–7.

48. Bagga HS, Tasian GE, Fisher PB, et al. Product related adult genitourinary injuries treated in United States Emergency Departments from 2002-2010. J Urol 2013;189(4):1362–8.

49. Bariol SV, Stewart GD, Smith RD, et al. An analysis of urinary tract trauma in Scotland: impact on management and resource needs. Surgeon 2005;3(1): 27–30.

50. Deibert CM, Spencer BA. The association between operative repair of bladder injury and improved survival: results from the National Trauma Data Bank. J Urol 2011;186(1):151–5.

51. Udekwu PO, Gurkin B, Oller DW. The use of computed tomography in blunt abdominal injuries. Am Surg 1996;62(1):56–9.

52. Bjurlin MA, Fantus RJ, Mellett MM, et al. Genitourinary injuries in pelvic fracture morbidity and mortality using the National Trauma Data Bank. J Trauma 2009;67(5):1033–9.

53. Gomez RG, Ceballos L, Coburn M, et al. Consensus statement on bladder injuries. BJU Int 2004;94(1):27–32.

54. Chapple C, Barbagli G, Jordan G, et al. Consensus statement on urethral trauma. BJU Int 2004;93(9): 1195–202.

55. Pereira BM, de Campos CC, Calderan TR, et al. Bladder injuries after external trauma: 20 years experience report in a population-based cross-sectional view. World J Urol 2012. [Epub ahead of print].

56. Tezval H, Tezval M, von Klot C, et al. Urinary tract injuries in patients with multiple trauma. World J Urol 2007;25(2):177–84.

57. Morey AF, Iverson AJ, Swan A, et al. Bladder rupture after blunt trauma: guidelines for diagnostic imaging. J Trauma 2001;51(4):683–6.

58. Avey G, Blackmore CC, Wessells H, et al. Radiographic and clinical predictors of bladder rupture in blunt trauma patients with pelvic fracture. Acad Radiol 2006;13(5):573–9.

59. Mendez LE. Iatrogenic injuries in gynecologic cancer surgery. Surg Clin North Am 2001;81(4): 897–923.

60. Levy BF, De Guara J, Willson PD, et al. Bladder injuries in emergency/expedited laparoscopic surgery in the absence of previous surgery: a case series. Ann R Coll Surg Engl 2012;94(3): e118–20.

61. Cass AS, Behrens F, Comfort T, et al. Bladder problems in pelvic injuries treated with external fixator and direct urethral drainage. J Trauma 1983; 23(1):50–3.

62. Bjornerem A, Tollan A. Intrauterine device–primary and secondary perforation of the urinary bladder. Acta Obstet Gynecol Scand 1997;76(4):383–5.

63. Mundy AR, Andrich DE. Pelvic fracture-related injuries of the bladder neck and prostate: their nature, cause and management. BJU Int 2010; 105(9):1302–8.

64. Mundy AR. Pelvic fracture injuries of the posterior urethra. World J Urol 1999;17(2):90–5.

65. Webster GD, Mathes GL, Selli C. Prostatomembranous urethral injuries: a review of the literature and a rational approach to their management. J Urol 1983;130(5):898–902.

66. Lowe MA, Mason JT, Luna GK, et al. Risk factors for urethral injuries in men with traumatic pelvic fractures. J Urol 1988;140(3):506–7.

67. Carter CT, Schafer N. Incidence of urethral disruption in females with traumatic pelvic fractures. Am J Emerg Med 1993;11(3):218–20.

68. Mundy AR, Andrich DE. Urethral trauma. Part I: introduction, history, anatomy, pathology, assessment and emergency management. BJU Int 2011; 108(3):310–27.

69. Koraitim MM. Pelvic fracture urethral injuries: the unresolved controversy. J Urol 1999;161(5): 1433–41.

70. Koraitim MM, Marzouk ME, Atta MA, et al. Risk 2factors and mechanism of urethral injury in pelvic fractures. Br J Urol 1996;77(6):876–80.

71. Basta AM, Blackmore CC, Wessells H. Predicting urethral injury from pelvic fracture patterns in male patients with blunt trauma. J Urol 2007; 177(2):571–5.

72. Song E, Trosseille X, Guillemot H. Side impact: influence of impact conditions and bone mechanical properties on pelvic response using a fracturable pelvis model. Stapp Car Crash J 2006;50: 75–95.

73. Breaud J, Baque P, Loeffler J, et al. Posterior urethral injuries associated with pelvic injuries in young adults: computerized finite element model creation and application to improve knowledge and prevention of these lesions. Surg Radiol Anat 2012;34(4):333–9.

74. Andrich DE, Mundy AR. The nature of urethral injury in cases of pelvic fracture urethral trauma. J Urol 2001;165(5):1492–5.

75. Cendron M, Whitmore KE, Carpiniello V, et al. Traumatic rupture of the corpus cavernosum: evaluation and management. J Urol 1990;144(4): 987–91.

76. Sant GR. Rupture of the corpus cavernosum of the penis. Arch Surg 1981;116(9):1176–8.

77. Al-Shaiji TF, Amann J, Brock GB. Fractured penis: diagnosis and management. J Sex Med 2009; 6(12):3231–40 [quiz: 3241].

78. Lynch TH, Martinez-Pineiro L, Plas E, et al. EAU guidelines on urological trauma. Eur Urol 2005; 47(1):1–15.

79. Saint S, Veenstra DL, Sullivan SD, et al. The potential clinical and economic benefits of silver alloy urinary catheters in preventing urinary tract infection. Arch Intern Med 2000;160(17):2670–5.

80. Kashefi C, Messer K, Barden R, et al. Incidence and prevention of iatrogenic urethral injuries. J Urol 2008;179(6):2254–7 [discussion: 2257–8].

81. Simhan J, Rothman J, Canter D, et al. Gunshot wounds to the scrotum: a large single-institutional 20-year experience. BJU Int 2012;109(11):1704–7.

82. Brandes SB, Buckman RF, Chelsky MJ, et al. External genitalia gunshot wounds: a ten-year experience with fifty-six cases. J Trauma 1995; 39(2):266–71 [discussion: 271–2].

83. McAninch JW, Kahn RI, Jeffrey RB, et al. Major traumatic and septic genital injuries. J Trauma 1984;24(4):291–8.

84. Lee JY, Cass AS, Streitz JM. Traumatic dislocation of testes and bladder rupture. Urology 1992;40(6): 506–8.

85. Phonsombat S, Master VA, McAninch JW. Penetrating external genital trauma: a 30-year single institution experience. J Urol 2008;180(1):192–5 [discussion: 195–6].

86. Mohr AM, Pham AM, Lavery RF, et al. Management of trauma to the male external genitalia: the usefulness of American Association for the Surgery of Trauma organ injury scales. J Urol 2003; 170(6 Pt 1):2311–5.

87. Cline KJ, Mata JA, Venable DD, et al. Penetrating trauma to the male external genitalia. J Trauma 1998;44(3):492–4.

88. Learch TJ, Hansch LP, Ralls PW. Sonography in patients with gunshot wounds of the scrotum: imaging findings and their value. AJR Am J Roentgenol 1995;165(4):879–83.

89. Ferguson GG, Brandes SB. Gunshot wound injury of the testis: the use of tunica vaginalis and polytetrafluoroethylene grafts for reconstruction. J Urol 2007;178(6):2462–5.

90. Cerwinka WH, Block NL. Civilian gunshot injuries of the penis: the Miami experience. Urology 2009; 73(4):877–80.

91. McAninch JW. Traumatic and reconstructive urology. Philadelphia: W.B. Saunders Company; 1996.

92. Aaronson DS, Shindel AW. U.S. national statistics on penile fracture. J Sex Med 2010;7(9):3226.

93. Morey AF, Metro MJ, Carney KJ, et al. Consensus on genitourinary trauma: external genitalia. BJU Int 2004;94(4):507–15.

94. Zargooshi J. Penile fracture in Kermanshah, Iran: report of 172 cases. J Urol 2000;164(2): 364–6.

95. Fergany AF, Angermeier KW, Montague DK. Review of Cleveland Clinic experience with penile fracture. Urology 1999;54(2):352–5.

96. Kramer AC. Penile fracture seems more likely during sex under stressful situations. J Sex Med 2011;8(12):3414–7.

97. Hudak SJ, Morey AF, Rozanski TA, et al. Battlefield urogenital injuries: changing patterns during the past century. Urology 2005;65(6):1041–6.

98. Paquette EL. Genitourinary trauma at a combat support hospital during Operation Iraqi Freedom: the impact of body armor. J Urol 2007;177(6): 2196–9 [discussion: 2199].

99. Marshall DF. Urogenital wounds in an evacuation hospital. J Urol 1946;55:119–32.

100. Serkin FB, Soderdahl DW, Hernandez J, et al. Combat urologic trauma in US military overseas

contingency operations. J Trauma 2010;69(Suppl 1): S175–8.

101. Waxman S, Beekley A, Morey A, et al. Penetrating trauma to the external genitalia in Operation Iraqi Freedom. Int J Impot Res 2009;21(2): 145–8.

102. Patel TH, Wenner KA, Price SA, et al. A U.S. Army Forward Surgical Team's experience in Operation Iraqi Freedom. J Trauma 2004;57(2):201–7.

103. Administration, NHTS. Traffic safety facts - research note. 2012. Available at: http://www-nrd. nhtsa.dot.gov/Pubs/811552.pdf. Accessed Januar 4, 2013.

104. Breaud J, Montoro J, Lecompte JF, et a Posterior urethral injuries associated with motc cycle accidents and pelvic trauma in adole cents: analysis of urethral lesions occurrir prior to a bony fracture using a computerize finite-element model. J Pediatr Urol 2013;9(1 62–70.

105. Youth violence: a report of the surgeon genera Psychiatr Serv 2001;52(3):399.

High-grade Renal Injuries

Radiographic Findings Correlated with Intervention for Renal Hemorrhage

Jeremy B. Myers, MD[a],*, William O. Brant, MD[a],
Joshua A. Broghammer, MD[b]

KEYWORDS

- Kidney • Trauma • Renal • Bleeding • Radiology • Model • Computed tomography

KEY POINTS

- Most high-grade renal injuries are managed conservatively. A key to successful nonoperative management is identifying those injuries that need intervention for continued renal hemorrhage.
- The American Association for the Surgery of Trauma (AAST) grading has been modified to decrease disparities in reporting of grades within the renal trauma literature, but there remains a broad categorization of risk for hemorrhage within grade 3 and 4 injuries.
- Specific radiographic parameters may serve as identifiers for patients at risk of continued renal hemorrhage.

BACKGROUND

Epidemiology of Kidney Injury

Renal injuries are relatively uncommon and are present in about 1% of patients hospitalized after traumatic injury.[1–3] Of all genitourinary trauma, however, the kidney is by far the most commonly injured organ in civilian institutions.[2,4] Extrapolations based on large renal trauma series estimate there to be an annual incidence of 245,000 traumatic renal injuries worldwide.[5] In large population-based studies, blunt injury is the leading mechanism of injury and accounts for between 81% and 95% of cases.[3–5] The mechanism of trauma can vary significantly, however, and single institutional series in urban centers demonstrate a much greater predominance of penetrating injury to the kidney.[6] Although the incidence of renal trauma is lower compared with other solid organ injuries regardless of the mechanism, these injuries can be associated with life-threatening complications of which renal hemorrhage is the most acute and dramatic.

Conservative Management of High-grade Injuries

Multiple studies have shown that high-grade renal trauma can be successfully managed in most cases conservatively.[7] This is true even in cases of penetrating trauma in patients that do not require laparotomy for other abdominal injuries, have undergone appropriate radiologic imaging, and have adequate renal injury staging.[8] The absolute indications for renal exploration are life-threatening hemorrhage from renovascluar injury; ureteropelvic junction avulsion; and urinoma unresponsive to minimally invasive procedures (ureteral stenting or perinephric drainage). The relative indications for exploration are laparotomy

Disclosures: The authors have no conflicts of interest or pertinent disclosures related to this article.
[a] Department of Surgery, The Center for Reconstructive Urology and Men's Health, University of Utah, Salt Lake City, UT, USA; [b] Department of Urology, University of Kansas Medical Center, Kansas City, KS, USA
* Corresponding author. Department of Surgery, University of Utah, 30 North 1900 East, Room #3B420, Salt Lake City, UT 84132.
E-mail address: jeremy.myers@hsc.utah.edu

for other abdominal injuries, concomitant pancreatic[9] or bowel injury,[10] and large devascularized segments of kidney.[11]

The importance of nonoperative management of renal injury is avoiding laparotomy and more importantly avoiding iatrogenic or unnecessary nephrectomy. At trauma centers with interest in renal trauma, nephrectomy is rare and reserved for renovascular injuries.[12] However, nationally studies have shown that the most common operation in the management of renal trauma remains nephrectomy.[1,2] In series where nonoperative management has been rigorously adopted, nephrectomy in high-grade renal trauma has dropped and proportionally renal salvage has risen.[13,14] It is intuitive and actually observed that after trauma nephrectomy renal function is halved,[15] although it is debated whether this leads to worse outcomes.[16] Despite this debate, it is obvious to any trauma surgeon that unnecessary nephrectomy in the setting of severely traumatized patients is harmful.

Because the most common management of renal injury remains nephrectomy,[17] conservative management of renal injuries, often with angioembolization when feasible, has been shown to decrease the rate of nephrectomy and increase renal salvage.

CURRENT GRADING OF RENAL INJURY

The American Association for the Surgery of Trauma (AAST) organ injury severity scale is the gold standard for assessment of traumatic renal injuries since its inception in 1989,[18] and it has been shown by multiple studies to provide excellent prognostic information.[19,20] The AAST grading scale, however, is very broad and there is a large spectrum of risk for complications, such as renal hemorrhage within AAST grade 3 and 4 injuries. In addition, there is significant discrepancy in grading between AAST grade 4 and 5 injuries within the literature. One reason this grading subjectivity arises is because of the ill-defined AAST grade 5 "shattered kidney." Many severe grade 4 injuries are categorized as grade 5 injuries because of this designation of "shattered kidney."

Modifications of AAST Grading

To eliminate this discrepant grading of renal injury prevalent throughout the trauma literature, Buckley and McAninch[21] recently proposed changes to the AAST grading system. The authors proposed that grade 5 injuries should include only those injuries that involved a main renal artery or renal vein injury and would cause in most cases total devascularization of the kidney by either renal hilar avulsion or an obstructive intimal arterial

flap (**Fig. 1**). Examples of grade 4 and 5 injuries with the modified AAST grading system, referred to by the authors as the revised Renal Injury Staging Classification (RISC), are illustrated in **Fig. 2**.

Adopting the revised RISC means that most injuries that demonstrated any vascularized and viable kidney are designated as a grade 4 injury. These changes expand the breadth of grade 4 injuries and also increase the spectrum of hemorrhage risk in grade 4 injury, the subject of this article. It is very important to understand the discrepancies in the reported outcomes of high grade renal injury within the literature to interpret the results from published series including prognostic nomograms and models.

Although the revised RISC encourages uniform reporting and a greater ability to compare results between studies, it does not increase the prognostic value of the system and the grade of renal injuries still remains very broad. When Buckley and McAninch[21] applied their proposed modifications to the large series from San Francisco General Hospital they found that only 2 of 52 patients with grade 5 injuries were downgraded to grade 4 and the changes made very little difference in the renal salvage rate (4.3% vs 4.2% in grade 5 injuries). However, this series was graded with a prejudice toward the modifications suggested in the recent article throughout its maintenance over the last four decades. In other series, such as Altman and colleagues,[22] where a salvage rate of grade 5 injuries was 46%, there is little doubt that reclassification of grade 5 injuries into the grade 4 category dramatically decreases the grade 5 renal salvage rates to make them more comparable with San Francisco General Hospital's series.

Thus, although these changes encompassed in the revised RISC may add uniformity within the literature they do little to increase the value of AAST grading to predict renal injuries that fail conservative management. Conversely, they act to broaden the definition of grade 4 injuries and the probable spectrum of clinical behavior of these injuries. Recognizing the wide spectrum of hemorrhage risk within grade 4 injuries, expanded by the revised RISC, highlights the importance of developing a predictive model in high-grade renal injury, especially given the greater contemporary role of conservative management of these injuries.

RADIOGRAPHIC PREDICTORS OF RENAL HEMORRHAGE

Four groups have looked at radiographic findings associated with renal hemorrhage after trauma.

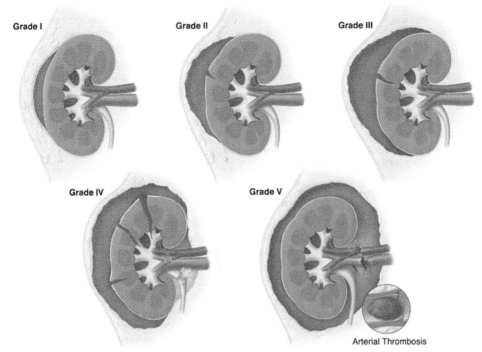

Fig. 1. Modified AAST grading intended to eliminate inconsistent reporting of grade 4 and 5 renal injuries. Grade [5] injuries, with this modification, would consist of those injuries with arterial thrombus or a renal hilar injury, such as renal hilar avulsion. The previous grade 5 "shattered kidney" is now referred to as a grade 4 injury if there [is a] vascularized kidney.

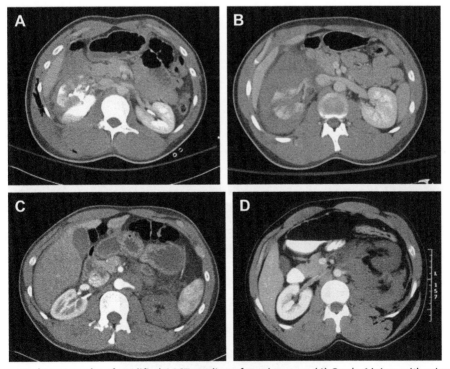

Fig. 2. Computed tomography of modified AAST grading of renal trauma. (*A*) Grade 4 injury with urinary extravasation. (*B*) Severe grade 4 laceration previously often categorized as grade 5 "shattered kidney." (*C*) Grade [5] injury with intimal flap from deceleration injury. (*D*) Grade 5 renal artery hilar avulsion. (*Courtesy of* Dr Jack McAninch, San Francisco General Hospital, San Francisco, CA.)

The first study, by Dugi and colleagues,[23] was reported from Parkland Hospital in 2010. Their patient population included 102 patients with grade 3 and 4 renal trauma, which was caused by blunt trauma in greater than 90% of cases. In patients with AAST grade 3 and 4 blunt renal injuries, they proposed three imaging characteristics that were independent risk factors associated with the need for intervention for bleeding. These included intravascular contrast extravasation; complex laceration (defined below); and perinephric hematoma greater than 3.5 cm.

These parameters were evaluated on the initial computed tomography (CT) scan, which was obtained on presentation to the emergency department. Intravascular contrast extravasation was identified during the arterial phase of the CT scan (**Fig. 3**). The location of the laceration was determined by drawing a line through the axis of the hilum of the kidney in cross-section and then drawing another line perpendicular to this, which transected the kidney into approximate quarters (see **Fig. 3**). Any laceration medial to this perpendicular line was classified as a medial laceration. Patients that had both a medial and a lateral laceration were classified as having a complex laceration. Perirenal hematoma distance was determined on the CT scan cross-section by the maximum measurement of the edge or rim of the hematoma from the capsule of the kidney on the CT scan cross-section (see **Fig. 3**).

The three risk factors in this study were all significantly independently associated with need for intervention for hemorrhage. Intravascular contrast extravasation, a complex laceration, and a perirenal hematoma distance greater than 3.5 cm increased the odds of intervention for hemorrhage by 13.8, 8.4, and 10, respectively. The authors then assigned 1 point to each of these risk factors and determined a "renal trauma risk score" with possible score of 0 to 3 points. They found that patients with 0 or 1 points had a risk of intervention for renal hemorrhage of 7% versus 67% in patients with 2 or 3 points. Overall, 18 of the 102 patients required intervention for hemorrhage (8 patients at AAST grade 3; 10 patients at AAST grade 4) and the overall predictive accuracy was 80% of their proposed model.

In a 2011 French study of angiographic intervention for renal hemorrhage after trauma, Charbit and colleagues[24] analyzed several CT scan criteria with regard to need for angiographic embolization (either selective or the entire kidney) after renal trauma. Their study included 52 patients that had

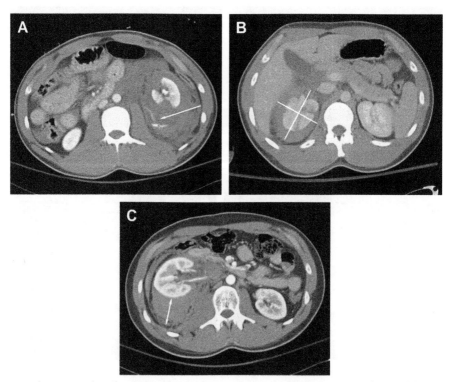

Fig. 3. Computed tomography of radiographic findings associated with intervention for renal hemorrhage. (A) Intravascular extravasation. (B) Both a medial and lateral laceration, classified as a complex laceration. (C) Measurement of a perirenal hematoma rim distance from the renal capsule to the rim of the hematoma.

AST grade 3 or higher injuries. The predominant mechanism was again blunt trauma in 89%. This study included only angiographic intervention in patients that were managed conservatively and, although all the patients had initial CT scan, five were excluded because they underwent nephrectomy or partial nephrectomy. Of the 52 patients managed conservatively that did not require operative management the authors analyzed the predictive value of intravascular extravasation, perirenal hematoma rim distance, laceration location, and discontinuity of Gerota fascia. All patients at their center who required greater than 2 units packed red blood cells and had intravascular extravasation or a large perirenal hematoma underwent angiography per their treatment protocol. They then tried to retrospectively correlate these and the other CT scan findings to the need for angioembolization.

The authors of this study were unable to correlate many of the CT scan findings with need for intervention with angioembolization. They were able, however, to define a patient group that absolutely did not need angiography and embolization as those that did not demonstrate intravascular extravasation and had a perirenal hematoma rim distance of less than 2.5 cm. This was found to be true despite some of these patients clinically demonstrating ongoing bleeding, which was attributed to other injuries.

In a set of studies from a Taiwanese group, several CT findings were studied to determine the need for angiographic intervention. The first of these studies in 2010 by Fu and colleagues[25] examined 26 patients undergoing angiography for blunt renal injury. Hemodynamically stable patients presenting with acute injury underwent CT scans as part of their trauma assessment. All patients with active contrast extravasation on CT underwent angiography and those with persistent bleeding then underwent embolization. The CT findings were reviewed retrospectively to look for predictors of the need for embolization. Of the 14 of 26 patients who underwent embolization, 79% had a disruption of Gerota fascia versus 2% in the nonembolization group. However, disruption of Gerota fascia was not found to be significant by Charbit and colleagues[24] in the French series.

In an update of their series, Lin and colleagues[26] looked at CT findings in those patients with renal trauma of AAST grade 3 or greater who underwent angiography. The angiography protocol was similar to the 2010 series. A total of 81 patients were included with 22 patients (27%) undergoing embolization. Contrast extravasation, extent of hematoma, and perirenal hematoma rim distance were all significant predictors of the need for embolization. Extent of hematoma was defined as extending down into the pelvis, across the right margin of the aorta for left-sided renal injuries, or extending across the left margin of the vena cava for right-sided renal injuries. The combination of contrast extravasation and extent of hematoma had the highest predictive value.

The final study originated from our own institution, the University of Utah.[17] In Utah, there are two adult level 1 trauma centers and the data were pooled from these centers. Penetrating trauma is rare in Utah (similar to the Parkland study, where only 5.8% of injuries had this mechanism)[23] and for this reason we excluded patients with this mechanism. We also excluded patients that were taken to the operating room immediately without a CT scan and patients that had grade 5 injuries as defined by the revisions recently suggested by Buckley and McAninch.[21] We found a total of 115 patients that met the inclusion criteria (blunt injury, AAST grade 3 or 4, CT scan done on presentation). We analyzed the three parameters defined by the Parkland Hospital group and found that intravascular extravasation and a perinephric hematoma rim distance greater than 3.5 cm both were associated with the need for intervention for hemorrhage by 16.4- and 8.4-fold, respectively. The location of laceration in the kidney, however, was not independently associated with intervention for renal hemorrhage, which was different than the findings from Parkland Hospital.

Our data also supported the Parkland Hospital's renal trauma risk score. We found that patients with 0 or 1 point had a risk of intervention of 2.9%, versus 18% and 50% in those patients that had 2 and 3 points, respectively. Our study was different in several important respects from the original Parkland study. We had a very low intervention rate of 7% (eight total patients) compared with 18% in the Parkland study.[23,24] The angiographic intervention rate was 20% in the French study and 27% in the Taiwanese study.[24,25] We hypothesized that this likely originated from differences in management regarding initial imaging and differences in threshold for treatment of ongoing hemorrhage. For instance, in the French study all 101 patients with renal trauma had a CT scan on presentation.[24] This is very different from our practice where patients with unstable hemodynamics and a positive focused abdominal sonogram for trauma examination are taken immediately for operative exploration without a CT scan. In our study 11 patients out of the 32 that were excluded had nephrectomy or partial nephrectomy. If these patients had undergone a CT scan before the operating room our intervention rate would have likely been much higher. Another practice variation that could easily account for differences in outcomes between the three studies is how tolerant centers and individual trauma surgeons are to hemorrhage. In the French study patients were taken for angiography if they needed greater than 2 units of packed red blood cells and had either intravascular extravasation or a "large" perirenal hematoma on their initial CT scan. The Taiwanese group had even less stringent criteria for angiography requiring only active vascular contrast extravasation on initial CT scan. Embolization was performed with any signs of bleeding on angiography regardless of transfusion requirements or hemodynamic status.[25,26] These criteria would be regarded as overly aggressive at many centers, and intuitively would lead to a much higher intervention rate than a more conservative strategy. Another example of different management strategies in regards to ongoing hemorrhage is that 44% (8 of 18) of patients in the Parkland study that required intervention had grade 3 injuries. This is dissimilar to our findings, where we found no patients with grade 3 injuries needed intervention. Another possible factor that could lead to the inconsistencies between the studies is differences in mechanism of injury. For instance, 21% of the patients in our series had sports-related injuries that often produce high-grade isolated renal injuries.[27] Patients with isolated renal injury could potentially tolerate more hemorrhage than those with multitrauma that are bleeding from many different sites.

DISCUSSION

All of the radiographic findings that have been explored as potential predictors of dangerous ongoing renal hemorrhage are independent of the AAST grade. These risk factors can be applied to an initial CT scan regardless of whether the AAST grade is correctly assigned. This is important because of the inconsistencies in grading patients with renal injury.[21] It is also important because in many trauma centers, including our own, correct genitourinary imaging after trauma can be difficult to obtain because of tertiary referral or ongoing management of other injuries. At our institution, only 73% of patients with high-grade renal injury or a perirenal fluid collection had appropriate imaging with an excretory phase CT scan.[28] The authors of the Parkland Hospital study, in their paper, proposed that AAST grading be modified to include a 4a and 4b category based on their renal trauma risk score. Those patients

with a renal trauma risk score with 0 to 1 points with a 7% risk of intervention would be classified as 4a and those patients with 2 to 3 points with a 67% risk of intervention would be classified as 4b

Clinical parameters have also been used successfully to define risk of intervention including renal exploration for hemorrhage independent of presenting imaging characteristics.[29,30] The ideal predictive model with reliable sensitivity and specificity would likely incorporate clinical and radiographic aspects of trauma patients' presentations to predict their hemorrhage risk and their clinical outcome. For instance an elderly patient with radiographic indicators of continued hemorrhage would likely need to be treated much more aggressively than a young patient with hemodynamic reserve. The same may be true of concomitant injuries. Patients that suffer from multiorgan trauma may not tolerate additional hemorrhage compared with patients with a solitary kidney injury, which is more often seen in sports-related accidents.[27]

A multi-institution study is needed that incorporates imaging characteristics at presentation and clinical factors, such as shock, presence of acidosis, comorbid state, concomitant injuries, injury severity score, initial hemoglobin, and ongoing transfusion requirements, among other factors to guide trauma surgeons about the need for interventions for continued renal hemorrhage.

SUMMARY

The success of the current movement toward nonoperative management of high-grade renal injuries would be strengthened with a precise and reproducible method of identifying patients at increased risk for renal hemorrhage. Failure of conservative management in the immediate setting is mostly from continued hemorrhage of a high-grade renal injury. A predictive nomogram or model would be invaluable in the setting of conservative management of renal injury and allow stratification of risk for continued renal hemorrhage. Trauma surgeons could then intervene with angioemobolization, nephrectomy, or partial nephrectomy if risk of hemorrhage was unacceptably high. A model or nomogram could also help guide referral to tertiary care centers or mandate a higher level of monitoring for hemorrhage in at-risk patients. Several radiographic findings have the potential of adding value in a model that predicts ongoing hemorrhage risk after high-grade renal trauma. Such a future model should also incorporate clinical patient characteristics, which would likely produce the most accurate predictive tool.

REFERENCES

1. Wright JL, Nathens AB, Rivara FP, et al. Renal and extrarenal predictors of nephrectomy from the National Trauma Data Bank. J Urol 2006;175(3):970–5.
2. Wessells H, Suh D, Porter JR, et al. Renal injury and operative management in the United States: results of a population-based study. J Trauma 2003;54(3):423–30.
3. Bariol SV, Stewart GD, Smith RD, et al. An analysis of urinary tract trauma in Scotland: impact on management and resource needs. Surgeon 2005;3(1):27–30.
4. Paparel P, N'Diaye A, Laumon B, et al. The epidemiology of trauma of the genitourinary system after traffic accidents: analysis of a register of over 43,000 victims. BJU Int 2006;97(2):338–41.
5. Santucci RA, Wessells H, Bartsch G, et al. Evaluation and management of renal injuries: consensus statement of the renal trauma subcommittee. BJU Int 2004;93(7):937–54.
6. Buckley JC, McAninch JW. Selective management of isolated and nonisolated grade IV renal injuries. J Urol 2006;176(6 Pt 1):2498–502 [discussion: 2502].
7. Broghammer JA, Fisher MB, Santucci RA. Conservative management of renal trauma: a review. Urology 2007;70(4):623–9.
8. Voelzke BB, McAninch JW. Renal gunshot wounds: clinical management and outcome. J Trauma 2009;66(3):593–600 [discussion: 600–1].
9. Rosen MA, McAninch JW. Management of combined renal and pancreatic trauma. J Urol 1994;152(1):22–5.
10. Wessells H, McAninch JW. Effect of colon injury on the management of simultaneous renal trauma. J Urol 1996;155(6):1852–6.
11. Moudouni SM, Patard JJ, Manunta A, et al. A conservative approach to major blunt renal lacerations with urinary extravasation and devitalized renal segments. BJU Int 2001;87(4):290–4.
12. Nash PA, Bruce JE, McAninch JW. Nephrectomy for traumatic renal injuries. J Urol 1995;153(3 Pt 1):609–11.
13. Hammer CC, Santucci RA. Effect of an institutional policy of nonoperative treatment of grades I to IV renal injuries. J Urol 2003;169(5):1751–3.
14. Moudouni SM, Hadj Slimen M, Manunta A, et al. Management of major blunt renal lacerations: is a nonoperative approach indicated? Eur Urol 2001;40(4):409–14.
15. McGonigal MD, Lucasv CE, Ledgerwood AM. The effects of treatment of renal trauma on renal function. J Trauma 1987;27(5):471–6.
16. Velmahos GC, Constantinou C, Gkiokas G. Does nephrectomy for trauma increase the risk of renal failure? World J Surg 2005;29(11):1472–5.
17. Hardee MJ, Lowrance W, Brant WO, et al. High grade renal injuries: application of Parkland Hospital's predictors of intervention for renal hemorrhage to a large series of patients with blunt renal trauma. J Urol 2013;189:1771–6.
18. Moore EE, Shackford SR, Pachter HL, et al. Organ injury scaling: spleen, liver, and kidney. J Trauma 1989;29(12):1664–6.
19. Santucci RA, McAninch JW, Safir M, et al. Validation of the American Association for the Surgery of Trauma organ injury severity scale for the kidney. J Trauma 2001;50(2):195–200.
20. Shariat SF, Roehrborn CG, Karakiewicz PI, et al. Evidence-based validation of the predictive value of the American Association for the Surgery of Trauma kidney injury scale. J Trauma 2007;62(4):933–9.
21. Buckley JC, McAninch JW. Revision of current American Association for the Surgery of Trauma Renal Injury grading system. J Trauma 2011;70(1):35–7.
22. Altman AL, Haas C, Dinchman KH, et al. Selective nonoperative management of blunt grade 5 renal injury. J Urol 2000;164(1):27–30 [discussion: 30–1].
23. Dugi DD III, Morey AF, Gupta A, et al. American Association for the Surgery of Trauma grade 4 renal injury substratification into grades 4a (low risk) and 4b (high risk). J Urol 2010;183(2):592–7.
24. Charbit J, Manzanera J, Millet I, et al. What are the specific computed tomography scan criteria that can predict or exclude the need for renal angioembolization after high-grade renal trauma in a conservative management strategy? J Trauma 2011;70(5):1219–27 [discussion: 1227–8].
25. Fu CY, Wu SC, Chen RJ, et al. Evaluation of need for angioembolization in blunt renal injury: discontinuity of Gerota's fascia has an increased probability of requiring angioembolization. Am J Surg 2010;199(2):154–9.
26. Lin WC, Lin CH, Chen JH, et al. Computed tomographic imaging in determining the need of embolization for high-grade blunt renal injury. J Trauma Acute Care Surg 2013;74(1):230–5.
27. Lloyd GL, Slack S, McWilliams KL, et al. Renal trauma from recreational accidents manifests different injury patterns than urban renal trauma. J Urol 2012;188(1):163–8.
28. Hardee MJ, Lowrance W, Stevens MH, et al. Process improvement in trauma: compliance with recommended imaging evaluation in the diagnosis of high grade renal injuries. J Trauma 2013;74:558–62.
29. Shariat SF, Trinh QD, Morey AF, et al. Development of a highly accurate nomogram for prediction of the need for exploration in patients with renal trauma. J Trauma 2008;64(6):1451–8.
30. McGuire J, Bultitude MF, Davis P, et al. Predictors of outcome for blunt high grade renal injury treated with conservative intent. J Urol 2011;185(1):187–91.

Damage Control Maneuvers for Urologic Trauma

Thomas G. Smith III, MD*, Michael Coburn, MD

KEYWORDS

- Damage control • Renal injury • Ureter injury • Bladder injury • Genital injury • Urine extravasation

KEY POINTS

- Damage control management of urologic injuries is performed in conjunction with the managing trauma team.
- Evaluation and management of genitourinary injuries in a damage control setting requires unconventional evaluation and surgical techniques because of the critical nature of this group of injured patients.
- Renal injury can often be expectantly managed because of containment of hemorrhage by normal fascial anatomy.
- Temporary urinary diversion through externalized tubes and catheters is acceptable and appropriate in the damage control setting.
- Complex genitourinary reconstructive surgery should be delayed until the patient is hemodynamically and metabolically stable for prolonged surgery.

INTRODUCTION

Damage control in the management of multiorgan trauma is a well-established principal in severely injured patients.[1] The underlying objective is patient survival at all costs. Typically, these patients are critically ill and an abbreviated laparotomy is performed to rapidly control life-threatening bleeding or injuries and the patient is temporarily closed and resuscitated in an intensive care unit setting. The clinical hallmark of patients requiring damage control is the triad of hypothermia, metabolic acidosis, and coagulopathy.[2,3] Since the term "damage control" was coined in 1993 this multiphase patient management strategy has been expanded to include nonabdominal trauma including thoracic, vascular, and neurosurgical.[1,4] The genitourinary organ system is also well suited to this style of management in this subgroup of patients.

Over the past 20 years, we have worked to select approaches to management of the urinary system that allow a common patient care philosophy with our trauma general surgeons. Many urologic injuries can be successfully managed with a planned delayed definitive management after initial hemodynamic control and resuscitation including certain renal, ureteral, bladder, urethral, and genital injuries. This article addresses injury selection, initial imaging and injury staging, initial management at damage control, options for definitive management of urologic trauma, and complications of urologic damage control. Additionally, a brief history of damage control and communication and interaction between the urologist the trauma surgeon are discussed.

Scott Department of Urology, Baylor College of Medicine, 1709 Dryden Street, 16th Floor, Houston, TX 77030, USA
* Corresponding author.
E-mail address: tgsmith@bcm.edu

Urol Clin N Am 40 (2013) 343–350
http://dx.doi.org/10.1016/j.ucl.2013.04.003

HISTORY OF DAMAGE CONTROL

Damage control is a systematic three-phase approach to management of critically injured patients presenting with the lethal clinical triad.[1] These patients typically undergo an initial abbreviated laparotomy to control life-threatening bleeding and fecal contamination (phase 1). This is followed by fluid resuscitation, correction of coagulopathy, and warming in the intensive care setting (phase 2). Then, after the patient is hemodynamically stable, they are returned to the operating room for definitive management of abdominal injuries and closure of the abdominal wall (phase 3). The evaluation of damage control began in the 1980s with the publication of multiple series evaluating a subset of critical patients with severe abdominal injuries.[5–8] Before this, the traditional concept was that an injured patient is evaluated in the emergency department and is taken to the operating room for a definitive procedure and the abdomen closed. In the 1980s, Feliciano and Mattox began to evaluate abdominal packing for severe liver injuries.[5,7,9] In a series of 300 consecutive abdominal gunshot wounds, they noted that survival in this group was worse in patients who developed the triad of acidosis, hypothermia, and coagulopathy.[9] Four years later, Burch and colleagues[10] described an abbreviated laparotomy in 200 patients with this same triad and noted a survival rate of 33%. The term damage control was coined in 1993 by Rotondo and coworkers[1] after their evaluation of 46 patients, 24 treated with abbreviated laparotomy, and found a survival benefit in patients with significant vascular and multiple visceral injuries. Since that time, damage control has continued to evolve as a major trauma management strategy for critically injured patients and has been applied in the civilian and military settings.[11–15]

GENERAL MANAGEMENT ISSUES
Emergency Department

Evaluation of the urinary system for injury has improved over time so that well-defined indications exist for examination, imaging, and laboratory study of these patients.[16,17] In general, all hemodynamically stable patients with gross hematuria or those patients with blunt or penetrating mechanism, microscopic hematuria, and an episode of hypotension (defined as systolic blood pressure of <90 mm Hg) require contrast-enhanced imaging.[17–20] In most modern trauma centers the preferred imaging technique is cross-sectional imaging by computed tomography.[16] In those patients who are not hemodynamically stable, imaging studies might not be feasible because often these individuals are rapidly transported to the operating room. Although desirable, confirmation of two functional kidneys preoperatively is not always possible in these settings.

Interaction with the trauma service is beneficial for deciding the urgency and necessity of imaging, facilitating the completion and performance of these studies when necessary, and placing and evaluating urinary drainage catheters. We have found that close preoperative collaboration with the trauma surgery team has facilitated the development of preoperative imaging protocols and streamlined intraoperative evaluation and management of urologic injuries.

Communication

In patients with multisystem trauma, successful management demands frequent and effective communication between various entities, especially between the teams of surgical specialties managing these patients. This is especially true in the damage control patient because their overall survival is lower as a result of the frequent triad of hypotension, hypothermia, and coagulopathy.[21,2]

The optimal time for consultation of surgical subspecialties by the trauma surgery service is "as soon as possible," irrespective of need for initial support. In our hospital, we are routinely notified in instances of penetrating trauma when the patient has gross hematuria while the patient is still being evaluated in the shock room. When notified at this stage, we can participate in the entire sequence of urinary system evaluation and management from initial recommendations for radiologic studies through possible surgical treatment. Furthermore, we are able to rapidly assist with drainage or diversion of the urinary system and discuss expected outcomes caused by delaying definitive management of the urinary system injuries. Although the trauma service ultimately controls patient management decisions, we believe that our early input allows for more complete patient care and improvement in outcomes in these critically injured patients.

Intraoperative Evaluation

In patients taken emergently to the operating room multiple options exist for evaluation. The "one-shot" intravenous urogram performed in the operating room provides basic information before intervention, namely the presence or absence of bilateral nephrograms.[23,24] One caveat in this setting is that a hypotensive patient may not have the intravascular volume or pressure to filter enough contrast through the collecting system to reate a nephrogram. A second, less conventional, option is to administer a vital dye, such as methylene blue or indigo carmine, intravenously and atraumatically occlude the ureter of the injured kidney.[25] Contralateral function can be confirmed with the collection of discolored urine in the catheter collection bag.

Injuries to the lower urinary tract should not delay urgent intervention when ongoing blood loss creates concern for patient survival. Evaluation of the urethra and bladder can readily be performed in the operating room after significant hemorrhage has been controlled. In patients with suspected urethral injury, options for intraoperative evaluation include cystoscopy or retrograde urethrogram after abdominal exploration. These evaluations should be performed before catheter insertion. The bladder can be evaluated by exploration and bladder distention with retrograde infusion of vital dye or with static stress cystogram after abdominal exploration and control of hemorrhage.

External genital injury is rarely life threatening and does not require preoperative evaluation in the unstable patient. Key considerations are control of hemorrhage with pressure dressing or clamping and suture ligation of bleeding vessels intraoperatively. Hemorrhage control can be performed either concomitantly with abdominal exploration or after life-threatening issues have been addressed.

Intraoperative Hemorrhage

Significant sources of bleeding within the genitourinary system include kidney, bladder, urethra, and genitalia. The specific management of organ-specific injury is discussed later; however, several important considerations merit special mention. Typically, retroperitoneal bleeding in the kidney is confined within Gerota's fascia or the perirenal fascia and can be left undisturbed. Indications for exploration include pulsatile retroperitoneal hematoma or ongoing bleeding through or around the perirenal fascia. Bladder hemorrhage manifests in two forms: extravesical or intravesical. Extravesical hemorrhage can occur into either the pelvis or abdominal cavity by laceration of the perivesical blood vessels or the detrusor muscle. Intravesical hemorrhage occurs from mucosal or detrusor laceration and can cause rapid, profuse gross hematuria. With extravesical hemorrhage, rapid suture ligation of bleeding or perivesical packing with laparotomy pads for control may be necessary. For intravesical hemorrhage, temporary hemorrhage control can be facilitated by catheter occlusion and clot tamponade with correction

or repair after the patient is stable. Genital bleeding is usually controlled with suture ligation, but definitive complex genital reconstruction often requires a future trip to the operating room.

Uncontrolled Urinary Extravasation

Although desirable, early urinary control is important but lower priority in the order of patient management issues. In contrast to uncontrolled fecal contamination, which can result in early sepsis, urine is typically sterile and does not pose this risk. However, ongoing urinary extravasation does create tissue irritation and can cause perinephric, retroperitoneal, peritoneal, or pelvic inflammation.[26] Because many techniques of temporary abdominal closure involve vacuum dressing or closed suction drains, often much of the extravasated urine is removed. Additionally, many options for temporary urinary diversion exist that can be rapidly implemented on either the initial exploration or at future surgery. This allows for definitive repair to be delayed or deferred until the patient is hemodynamically stable and reconstructive surgery is appropriate. For upper-tract injuries, an externalized stent can be quickly placed and provide thorough urinary diversion. In lower-tract injuries, such as significant bladder injuries, which cannot be quickly repaired, ureteral diversion stents prevent or lessen pelvic or abdominal urinary extravasation and subsequent inflammatory response.

MANAGEMENT OF SPECIFIC ORGAN INJURIES
Renal Injury

Our approach to intraoperative evaluation and management of renal injuries begins with an assessment of the patient's hemodynamic stability and discussion with the operating trauma service about management goals. Often, a patient undergoing abbreviated laparotomy and damage control management has limited preoperative radiologic evaluation. In these cases, decision-making is based on operative findings and available adjunctive studies. Most renal injuries are amenable to a damage control approach with the exceptions being expanding or pulsatile hematoma and ongoing uncontained hemorrhage. We have found that expectant management is successful and appropriate in those patients who are not hemodynamically stable enough to undergo the necessary reconstruction in salvageable injuries.[27–29] Additionally, it is common practice in urologic trauma patient management to observe and monitor high-grade renal injuries from blunt mechanism.[27–30] Our approach in damage control patients is to evaluate but not necessarily explore a confined retroperitoneal hematoma or hemorrhage. Delayed formal exploration and reconstruction can then be performed in a fully resuscitated and more stable patient.

In those patients with penetrating injuries, the injury is often apparent based on the site of retroperitoneal penetration.[31] Blunt injuries can be more challenging because the retroperitoneal fascia is often intact and without the benefit of preoperative imaging, the exact location of the injury is more difficult to ascertain. In these patients, evaluation of the hematoma is paramount in deciding which patients to explore. We have observed that retroperitoneal hematomas requiring exploration are relatively easy to identify, usually indicate renal pedicle injury, and are a life-threatening emergency. The most difficult patients to manage are those with an intimal arterial disruption causing vascular occlusion. In those patients without preoperative imaging, the surgeon must decide if the injury warrants exploration and if the patient is stable enough to undergo evaluation and repair of the arterial injury. Often, in patients undergoing abbreviated laparotomy, the patient's condition dictates that unilateral arterial intimal repair be delayed, especially in the presence of a normal contralateral kidney. In these cases, prolonged warm ischemia usually results in irreparable damage and renal loss.

Further retroperitoneal exploration can be performed without disturbing the contained renal hematoma. Central retroperitoneal hematomas (zone 1) are concerning for vascular injuries, namely the aorta and vena cava. If an injury to these structures is suspected, the trauma surgeon can enter the retroperitoneum and leave the confined renal hematoma undisturbed within the perinephric fascia. If the perirenal fascia is violated and renal cortical bleeding is noted, packing the renal fossa tightly with laparotomy pads can salvage the kidney in an unstable patient. At a future operation, the packs can be removed, the wound irrigated, and the injury repaired in the appropriately selected patient.[25,32]

A risk of damage control management is that ongoing or even life-threating hemorrhage can occur from the injured kidney while the patient is resuscitated, warmed, and awaits re-exploration and repair. However, our experience has shown that this is not a frequent occurrence and careful monitoring, as in all patients undergoing damage control, is sufficient. In the damage control setting, major renal parenchymal injury can result in urinary extravasation that is difficult to control without significant reconstructive efforts. Our usual approach is to begin with external drainage and plan for management at a future operation. In general, a

brief period of controlled local urinary extravasation is unlikely to result in a significant adverse event or impact overall recovery of the patient.

During phase 2 in the damage control process, which is usually a period of 48 to 72 hours, suspected renal injuries identified in the first laparotomy are staged. In most patients, we obtain cross-sectional imaging with contrast-enhanced computed tomography scans to identify injuries and select patients for subsequent operation and reconstruction or continued expectant management with no plan for operative intervention.[16,3] Identifying renal injuries that are appropriate for nonoperative management allows the trauma surgery team to concentrate on other critical injuries and does not expose the patient to the potential morbidity of unnecessary renal surgery. The most important point is to fully stage unknown or suspected injuries.

In select patients, adjunct imaging including arteriography may be appropriate. In these situations, arteriography can be diagnostic and therapeutic for renal, vascular, or solid organ injury. In some injured patients, angioembolization is an appropriate and less morbid treatment especially during phase 2 of damage control management. However, emerging data show an overuse of angioembolization in the management of renal injury based on grade of the injury.[33] An individualized approach to the selection of operative versus angiographic control of delayed renal hemorrhage is important and should be based on factors including level of radiologic expertise available, other nonurologic indications, severity of renal injury, and stability of the patient.

In patients who require delayed definitive operative management, the concepts and operative steps are similar to other renal trauma management.[23] We believe that initial hilar control is important and thus the hilum is initially accessed to provide for arterial and venous control. We have also developed an alternative method of vascular control that does not involve individual control of the renal artery and vein.[19,25] In this technique, vascular control is obtained by bluntly dissecting along the plane of the psoas muscle fascia, adjacent to the great vessels, and directly placing a vascular pedicle clamp on the renal hilum. We have found this particularly helpful in instances where significant or rapid bleeding is noted. Regardless of the method of vascular control used, it is important to avoid unnecessary nephrectomy because of diffuse bleeding from inadequate control of the renal hilum. After vascular control, the kidney is mobilized, the perirenal fascia opened, and the hematoma is evacuated. After the kidney is adequately exposed, the injury is debrided and definitive repair is performed. We believe that ureteral stenting or nephrostomy diversion should be strongly considered after delayed reconstruction because of the increased risk of postoperative urinary extravasation compared with primary repairs.

Ureteral Injury

Damage control management of ureteral injury is readily applicable for many reasons.[34,35] Primarily, the risk of bleeding secondary to a ureteral injury is minimal and outweighed by more pressing concerns with other injuries. Additionally, there are many available options for urinary diversion which can be rapidly implemented that preserve tissue quality and anatomic relationships. Finally, ureteral reconstruction can be a challenging and time-consuming endeavor.[35] Depending on the level of ureteral injury and the status of surrounding tissues, temporary urinary diversion or adjuvant measures may be the best management option when the patient is unstable and resuscitation in the intensive care unit is necessary.

A ureteral injury can be diverted using any number of small, hollow medical tubes to intubate the ureteral lumen and externalize the open end of the selected tube. Our preference is to use "single-J" stents (**Fig. 1**), commonly used in elective urinary diversion procedures; however, a Cordis catheter, central line, or feeding tube can be used with equal efficacy if a specific stent is not available. Regardless of diversion method, it is

important to use a guide wire to ensure that the device travels proximally into the renal pelvis. We secure the stent or tube to the proximal ureter using a 3-0 silk suture and only compress a minimal amount of ureteral tissue (1–2 mm). This prevents migration or dislodgement of the stent and at the same time preserves ureteral tissue for future repair. The distal end of the stent is externalized through a stab incision in the abdominal wall and secured to the skin, after which a drainage bag is placed. With the urine diverted in this fashion, renal output can be monitored until the patient can safely return to the operating room for definitive repair. If the stent becomes occluded with blood clots or debris, the free lumen can be gently irrigated with saline until drainage resumes. If there is any question as to the position of the stent, either plain radiographs or injection of contrast confirms the location of the proximal aspect of the stent. In cases of complete ureteral transection, we do not manipulate, ligate, or divert the distal end of the ureter. Usually, urinary reflux is not a concern in injured patients. If the distal ureter is manipulated or ligated this damages the tissue resulting in ureteral tissue loss and affects the future reconstruction of the ureter.

If the patient's condition does not allow for diversion as described previously or no appropriate tube or device is available, an option for management is proximal ureteral ligation with diversion of the urine by a nephrostomy tube typically placed postoperatively in the interventional radiology suite. The ureter can drain freely into the abdominal cavity, if necessary, with urinary drainage by an external drain or as part of the temporary abdominal closure. However, our preferred method of drainage and diversion is an intubated, externalized stent that allows for assessment of renal output and is easy to perform. The initial management of these injuries is certainly within the ability of the managing trauma service. We believe that early urologic consultation is important for evaluation in the initial laparotomy and planning purposes in future reconstructive surgeries.

In phase 3, the stable patient returns to the operating room for reconstruction. We re-evaluate the ureter at that setting to determine the appropriate reconstructive technique, typically either primary ureteroureterostomy (spatulated end-to-end anastomosis) or ureteroneocystostomy (reimplantation into the bladder).[35] The former is used for reconstruction of upper and select midureteral injuries and the latter is used for reconstruction of distal ureteral and select midureteral injuries or lower ureteral loss. Other reconstructive techniques may be required (Boari

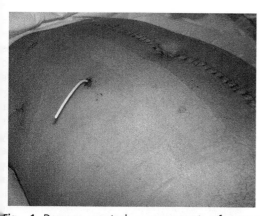

Fig. 1. Damage control management of upper ureteral laceration sustained from abdominal gunshot wound. A single-J stent is brought out for temporary urinary diversion. The patient was cold, unstable, and coagulopathic; bowel injuries were stapled off acutely. Delayed planned re-exploration with bowel and ureteral reconstruction was safely conducted the next day after vigorous resuscitation.

flap, ileal ureter, and so forth) but these are beyond the focus of this article. Again, use of stents and urinary diversion are encouraged because of the increased likelihood of postoperative anastomotic extravasation in the setting of delayed reconstruction. Furthermore, any injury or repair performed in proximity to an intestinal injury should have tissue separation with either omentum or other tissue interposition techniques (eg, peritoneum) to isolate any postoperative leaks and minimize these potential effects on the repair of nonurologic injuries.

Bladder

On occasion, a patient sustains pelvic trauma with bladder injury, regardless of mechanism, and is too hemodynamically unstable to undergo primary bladder repair. In blunt trauma, this may occur in patients with complex bladder rupture related to severe pelvic fracture and pelvic bleeding. In penetrating trauma, these patients may have multiple pelvic gunshot wounds or a high-velocity missile injury with injury to other pelvic organs (colon) or devastating vascular injuries. Management of extraperitoneal bladder injury from blunt mechanism is well described and most patients managed in this fashion recover completely.[36,37] Others have described management of select penetrating injuries to the bladder, which are completely extraperitoneal with simple catheter drainage.[38] It is appropriate to temporarily drain the bladder with a transurethral Foley catheter or suprapubic cystostomy catheter in the patient undergoing abbreviated laparotomy. For extensive bladder injury, no direct bladder drainage by catheter adequately drains the urine and thus ureteral stents may be passed into the ureteral orifices bilaterally and externalized to divert the urinary output of the kidneys temporarily.

We have used multiple techniques for urinary diversion in unstable patients with complex bladder injuries. The technique described previously is efficient in hemodynamically unstable patients with concomitant bladder and pelvic injuries. Alternatively, we have used a closed suction drain placed in proximity of the bladder and initially left the drain off suction (to allow for a pelvic hematoma to form) and then began suction after coagulopathy and fluid resuscitation has been initiated.

Urethra

Most urologists are familiar with the damage control techniques used in posterior urethral injuries.[37,39] In these patients, a suprapubic cystostomy tube is placed for initial urinary diversion and then elective repair is completed weeks or months after the initial injury. In patients with blunt and penetrating posterior urethral injury, we continue to consider early endoscopic realignment after the patient has been fully resuscitated and returns to the operating room. However, regardless of the secondary approach, the management of posterior urethral injuries follows the general principals of damage control management, which is rapid diversion of the urine as a temporizing measure and re-evaluation of the stable patient. Penetrating posterior injuries may require rapid control of bleeding with suture ligation and packing before urinary diversion. We do not believe that significant manipulation of posterior urethral injuries is indicated in the unstable patient and in these injuries the role of the urologist is to obtain bladder access for urinary diversion in the most expeditious and least morbid approach possible. Most are amenable to successful delayed, single-stage anastomotic repair (Fig. 2).

In anterior urethral injuries, patients undergoing abbreviated laparotomy typically either sustain complex or multiple penetrating injuries or complex pelvic or perineal trauma. In those with penetrating injury, suture ligation for control of urethral bleeding may be necessary. Otherwise, the approach in these patients is urinary drainage either with transurethral or suprapubic cystostomy tube drainage and delayed definitive reconstruction.

External Genitalia

Injuries to the external genitalia are rarely life-threatening and thus, damage control is appropriate

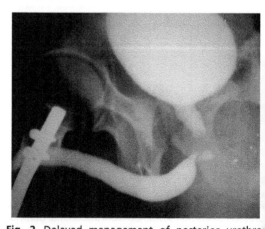

Fig. 2. Delayed management of posterior urethral gunshot wound. Combined retrograde urethrogram and cystogram reveal short obliterative bulbomembranous defect, successfully reconstructed by elective posterior urethroplasty involving excision with primary anastomosis.

these injuries.[37,40,41] In multisystem trauma, initial management is compression with pressure dressings and then wound irrigation and limited debridement to preserve tissue for future reconstructive surgery. Arterial bleeding may require suture ligation but these vessels are readily identified in the wound and this step can be performed during the abbreviated laparotomy. Our approach is to limit indiscriminate cauterization and excessive tissue debridement at damage control laparotomy. Determining which tissues are viable long-term is difficult prior to patient resuscitation. Wound vac dressings are an excellent adjunctive measure to be considered for devastating genital skin loss injuries.

COMPLICATIONS OF DAMAGE CONTROL MANAGEMENT FOR UROLOGIC INJURIES

In our experience, complications from delayed repair of renal, ureteral, and bladder injuries are more common than in patients undergoing repair and reconstruction at initial injury presentation. We have two hypotheses about this observation. The delicate urinary tissues become inflamed and edematous following injury making repair more challenging. Injuries that require deferred management may represent more complex wounds and thus are more technically difficult to repair. Based on this, we more frequently use stents and urinary diversion, tissue interposition when possible, and early adoption of antibiotics therapy, especially in those patients with initial external diversion of urine.

SUMMARY

Damage control management of urologic injuries is a technique borrowed from general trauma surgical principles but applicable to the entire urinary system. The objective is to restore normal genitourinary anatomy and function by temporizing ongoing derangements while the critically injured patient is resuscitated and warmed. Often, unconventional evaluation and management is necessary in the phase 1 surgery of damage control and proven urologic techniques can be implemented in the phase 3 surgery. The most important aspects of damage control surgery from the urologist's perspective are communication of the initial injuries and future management plans and availability to assist the trauma service with ongoing patient evaluation. Ongoing outcomes analyses are required to evaluate the best management strategies and identify novel techniques that lessen complications and promote return of optimal genitourinary function.

REFERENCES

1. Rotondo MF, Schwab CW, McGonigal MD, et al. Damage control: an approach for improved survival in exsanguinating penetrating abdominal injury. J Trauma 1993;35(3):375–82 [discussion: 382–3].
2. Bernabei AF, Levison MA, Bender JS. The effects of hypothermia and injury severity on blood loss during trauma laparotomy. J Trauma 1992;33(6):835–9.
3. Jurkovich GJ, Greiser WB, Luterman A, et al. Hypothermia in trauma victims: an ominous predictor of survival. J Trauma 1987;27(9):1019–24.
4. Chovanes J, Cannon JW, Nunez TC. The evolution of damage control surgery. Surg Clin North Am 2012; 92(4):859–75, vii–viii.
5. Feliciano DV, Mattox KL, Jordan GL Jr. Intraabdominal packing for control of hepatic hemorrhage: a reappraisal. J Trauma 1981;21(4):285–90.
6. Feliciano DV, Mattox KL, Jordan GL Jr, et al. Management of 1000 consecutive cases of hepatic trauma (1979-1984). Ann Surg 1986;204(4):438–45.
7. Feliciano DV, Mattox KL, Burch JM, et al. Packing for control of hepatic hemorrhage. J Trauma 1986;26(8): 738–43.
8. Cue JI, Cryer HG, Miller FB, et al. Packing and planned reexploration for hepatic and retroperitoneal hemorrhage: critical refinements of a useful technique. J Trauma 1990;30(8):1007–11 [discussion: 1011–3].
9. Feliciano DV, Burch JM, Spjut-Patrinely V, et al. Abdominal gunshot wounds. An urban trauma center's experience with 300 consecutive patients. Ann Surg 1988;208(3):362–70.
10. Burch JM, Ortiz VB, Richardson RJ, et al. Abbreviated laparotomy and planned reoperation for critically injured patients. Ann Surg 1992;215(5): 476–83 [discussion: 483–4].
11. Holcomb JB, Champion HR. Military damage control. Arch Surg 2001;136(8):965–7.
12. Holcomb JB, Helling TS, Hirshberg A. Military, civilian, and rural application of the damage control philosophy. Mil Med 2001;166(6):490–3.
13. Talbert S, Trooskin SZ, Scalea T, et al. Packing and re-exploration for patients with nonhepatic injuries. J Trauma 1992;33(1):121–4 [discussion: 124–5].
14. Walker ML. The damage control laparotomy. J Natl Med Assoc 1995;87(2):119–22.
15. Hirshberg A, Wall MJ Jr, Mattox KL. Planned reoperation for trauma: a two year experience with 124 consecutive patients. J Trauma 1994;37(3):365–9.
16. Alsikafi NF, Rosenstein DI. Staging, evaluation, and nonoperative management of renal injuries. Urol Clin North Am 2006;33(1):13–9, v.
17. Santucci RA, Wessells H, Bartsch G, et al. Evaluation and management of renal injuries: consensus statement of the renal trauma subcommittee. BJU Int 2004;93(7):937–54.

18. Carroll PR, McAninch JW. Operative indications in penetrating renal trauma. J Trauma 1985;25(7): 587–93.

19. Coburn M. Genitourinary trauma. In: Moore EE, Feliciano DV, Mattox KL, editors. Trauma, vol., 6th edition. New York: McGraw-Hill; 2008. p. 789–826.

20. Shariat SF, Trinh QD, Morey AF, et al. Development of a highly accurate nomogram for prediction of the need for exploration in patients with renal trauma. J Trauma 2008;64(6):1451–8.

21. Hirshberg A, Mattox KL. Damage control in trauma surgery. Br J Surg 1993;80(12):1501–2.

22. Morris JA Jr, Eddy VA, Blinman TA, et al. The staged celiotomy for trauma. Issues in unpacking and reconstruction. Ann Surg 1993;217(5):576–84 [discussion: 584–6].

23. Master VA, McAninch JW. Operative management of renal injuries: parenchymal and vascular. Urol Clin North Am 2006;33(1):21–31, v–vi.

24. Santucci R, Doumanian LR. Upper urinary tract trauma. In: Wein AJ, Kavoussi LR, Novick AC, et al, editors. Campbell-Walsh urology, vol. 2, 10th edition. Philadelphia: Elsevier-Saunders; 2012. p. 1169–89.

25. Coburn M. Damage control for urologic injuries. Surg Clin North Am 1997;77(4):821–34.

26. Husmann DA, Gilling PJ, Perry MO, et al. Major renal lacerations with a devitalized fragment following blunt abdominal trauma: a comparison between nonoperative (expectant) versus surgical management. J Urol 1993;150(6):1774–7.

27. Hammer CC, Santucci RA. Effect of an institutional policy of nonoperative treatment of grades I to IV renal injuries. J Urol 2003;169(5):1751–3.

28. Broghammer JA, Fisher MB, Santucci RA. Conservative management of renal trauma: a review. Urology 2007;70(4):623–9.

29. Santucci RA, Fisher MB. The literature increasingly supports expectant (conservative) management of renal trauma: a systematic review. J Trauma 2005; 59(2):493–503.

30. Alsikafi NF, McAninch JW, Elliott SP, et al. Nonoperative management outcomes of isolated urinary extravasation following renal lacerations due external trauma. J Urol 2006;176(6 Pt 1):2494–7.

31. Wessells H, McAninch JW, Meyer A, et al. Criteria for nonoperative treatment of significant penetrating renal lacerations. J Urol 1997;157(1):24–7.

32. Chaabouni MN, Bittard M. Application of a peri-renal prosthesis (Vicryl mesh) in the conservative treatment of multiple ruptured kidney fragments. Ann Urol (Paris) 1996;30(2):61–3 [discussion: 64] [in French].

33. Hotaling JM, Sorensen MD, Smith TG III, et al. Analysis of diagnostic angiography and angioembolization in the acute management of renal trauma using a national data set. J Urol 2011;185(4):1316–20.

34. Best CD, Petrone P, Buscarini M, et al. Traumatic ureteral injuries: a single institution experience validating the American Association for the Surgery of Trauma-Organ Injury Scale grading scale. J Urol 2005;173(4):1202–5.

35. Brandes S, Coburn M, Armenakas N, et al. Diagnosis and management of ureteric injury: an evidence based analysis. BJU Int 2004;94(3):277–89.

36. Gomez RG, Ceballos L, Coburn M, et al. Consensus statement on bladder injuries. BJU Int 2004;94(1): 27–32.

37. Morey AF, Dugi DD. Genital and lower urinary tract trauma. In: Wein AJ, Kavoussi LR, Novick AC, et al, editors. Campbell-Walsh Urology, vol 2, 10th edition. Philadelphia: Elsevier-Saunders; 2012. p. 2507–20.

38. Djakovic N, Plas E, Martinez-Pineiro L, et al. Guidelines of urological trauma. European Association of Urology; 2009. Available at: http://www.uroweb.org/gls/pdf/22_Urological_Trauma_LR%20II.pdf. Accessed December 15, 2012.

39. Chapple C, Barbagli G, Jordan G, et al. Consensus statement on urethral trauma. BJU Int 2004;93(9): 1195–202.

40. Morey AF, Metro MJ, Carney KJ, et al. Consensus on genitourinary trauma: external genitalia. BJU Int 2004;94(4):507–15.

41. van der Horst C, Martinez Portillo FJ, Seif C, et al. Male genital injury: diagnostics and treatment. BJU Int 2004;93(7):927–30.

Strategies for Open Reconstruction of Upper Ureteral Strictures

Richard B. Knight, MD[a],*, Steven J. Hudak, MD[b],
Allen F. Morey, MD[c]

KEYWORDS

• Ureter • Reconstruction • Stricture • Bladder flap • Ileal ureter

KEY POINTS

• The guiding surgical principle during ureteral reconstruction is creation of a tension-free, watertight anastomosis using absorbable sutures that is widely spatulated with preserved blood supply.
• Important factors when planning for ureteral reconstruction include length/location of the stricture, need for bowel interposition, and need to access the bladder.
• Urologists who repair proximal ureteral strictures should be familiar with ureteroureterostomy, transureteroureterostomy, downward nephropexy, ureterocalicostomy, bladder flap, psoas hitch, bowel interposition, and nephrectomy.

INTRODUCTION

Proximal ureteral strictures present a complex challenge to the urologist, often necessitating familiarity with a variety of surgical strategies for management. Because so many options exist for repair of the proximal ureteral stricture, consensus regarding optimal treatment can be elusive. The characteristics of each patient and surgeon's experience combine to determine the surgical plan. When considering the repair of a proximal ureteral stricture, the urologist should be familiar with the techniques listed in **Box 1**. The importance of understanding these surgical approaches is highlighted by the increased incidence of ureteral injury secondary to the advent of ureteroscopy and laparoscopy.[1]

Given the retroperitoneal location of the ureter, it is well protected from external trauma. It is therefore expected that ureteral trauma occurs in only 2.5% of all genitourinary injuries, most of which are caused by penetrating injury (61.5%–96.5%) within the proximal ureter (70%).[2–4] In the acute trauma setting, it may be necessary to delay definitive reconstruction of ureteral injuries until the patient is stable. This delay may warrant well-established temporary damage control maneuvers, such as externalized single-J ureteral catheter placement or ligation of the proximal ureter with postoperative placement of a nephrostomy tube.[5]

PREOPERATIVE EVALUATION

Numerous patient characteristics must be considered when deciding on the surgical approach to proximal ureteral strictures (**Box 2**). The importance of a thorough patient history and physical examination cannot be overemphasized.

Disclaimer: The opinions expressed in this document are solely those of the authors and do not represent an endorsement by or the views of the United States Air Force, the United States Army, the Department of Defense or the United States Government.

[a] Department of Urology, San Antonio Uniformed Services Health Education Consortium, 3851 Roger Brooke Drive, Fort Sam Houston, TX 78234, USA; [b] Department of Surgery, Urology Section, San Antonio Military Medical Center, 3851 Roger Brooke Drive, Fort Sam Houston, TX 78234, USA; [c] Department of Urology, UT Southwestern Medical Center, 5323 Harry Hines Boulevard, Dallas, TX 75390-9110, USA
* Corresponding author. Department of Urology, San Antonio Military Medical Center, 3851 Roger Brooke Drive, Fort Sam Houston, TX 78234.
E-mail address: richard_b_knight@yahoo.com

Box 1
Surgical techniques for proximal ureteral defect

Ureteroureterostomy

Transureteroureterostomy

Downward nephropexy

Ureterocalicostomy

Bladder flap

Psoas hitch

Bowel interposition

Renal autotransplantation

Nephrectomy

A preoperative urinalysis and urine culture are mandatory with antibiotics as indicated. Mechanical bowel preparation should be performed for any patient who may potentially undergo an intestinal substitution of the ureter.[6] In patients with intact bilateral kidneys, a functional study should be performed to establish differential renal function. Antegrade and/or retrograde ureterography are essential to determine the length and severity of the stricture. Excretory urography (nuclear or radiographic) is helpful in confirming obstruction in equivocal cases. If doubt remains regarding significant ureteral obstruction, a Whitaker test may be performed, although we have rarely resorted to this.

We prefer routinely removing ureteral stents before ureteral reconstruction, thus using a nephrostomy for renal drainage. Removal of ureteral stents allows for delineation of normal versus fibrotic luminal assessment. If the stent is retained

---

Box 2
Patient characteristics determining surgical approach

Number of previous failed endoscopic and/or open attempts

Length of stricture

Location of stricture

Function and drainage of each kidney

History of nephrolithiasis

Medical comorbidities

Life expectancy

History of malignancy

Previous radiation therapy

Bladder capacity

History of inflammatory bowel disease

---

before surgery, we have found that it may interfere with identification of the stricture.

SURGICAL PRINCIPLES

The guiding surgical principle during ureteral reconstruction is creation of a tension-free, watertight anastomosis using absorbable sutures that is widely spatulated with preserved blood supply, allowing good drainage to the bladder.[7,8] Maintaining the continuity of the urothelium (ie, avoiding intestinal interposition) is advocated whenever possible for reconstruction of the ureter.[9–11] The dissection of the nondiseased portions of the ureter should be minimized to avoid disrupting the ureteric adventitial sheath and its vascular supply. However, complete excision of the pathologic portions of the ureter is paramount to prevent recurrent strictures.[12]

The urothelial anastomosis may be wrapped with omentum, peritoneum, or perinephric fat to reduce the risk of leakage and improve the vascular supply. An omental flap is harvested by dissecting the omentum from the greater curvature of the stomach. The resulting omental flap obtains its blood supply from the right or left gastroepiploic vessels.[13,14]

Depending on the type of reconstruction, retroperitoneal and/or intraperitoneal drainage in combination with ureteral stent placement and bladder drainage are used routinely, but are not always performed.[13] A passive drain may be preferable to suction drainage to prevent negative pressure on the anastomotic suture line.[13] We prefer to use both drains and stents.

INCISION

Important factors when planning the incision and surgical approach for ureteral reconstruction include the length/location of the stricture, the need for bowel interposition, and the need to access the bladder. These factors also guide the decision to perform the reconstruction via an intraperitoneal or extraperitoneal approach. If limited proximal ureteral dissection is planned without accessing the bladder, a flank, Gibson, or pararectal incision may be used.[15] A midline incision is preferred for transureteroureterostomy or when the need for bowel interposition is anticipated.[16] However, optimal extraperitoneal exposure of the ipsilateral ureter and bladder may be accomplished through a modified Gibson incision that extends from the tip of the twelfth rib inferiorly in a lazy-S configuration toward the pubic symphysis.[17]

URETEROURETEROSTOMY

Ureteroureterostomy is the preferred reconstruction method for short proximal ureteral strictures

a tension-free anastomosis is possible. It is crit-
al to fully excise the strictured portion of the ure-
r until healthy epithelial edges are observed.[18]
he ureter is either transected obliquely (as initially
escribed by Bovee[19] in 1897) or spatulated for 10
• 15 mm to reduce the risk of anastomotic nar-
wing and subsequent stricture.[6,19] Anastomosis
performed with either interrupted or continuous
-0 or 5-0 absorbable suture.[20]

Numerous maneuvers may be necessary to pro-
de sufficient ureteral length for a tension-free
pair. If the renal pelvis is enlarged, it is possible
› achieve additional length by performing a
eineke-Mikulicz transverse incision of the superior
d medial renal pelvis with closure in a longitudinal
rientation.[21] The distance achieved with this ma-
euver is determined by the size of the renal pelvis
d the length of the pyelotomy. Renal mobilization
d downward nephropexy to the quadratus lum-
orum or psoas muscle have been shown to provide
n additional 4 cm of proximal ureteral length.[18]

Although historical reports showed high compli-
ation rates from ureteroureterostomy,[22] more
ontemporary series indicate long term patency
tes beyond 90% with low morbidity.[23,24]

RANSURETEROURETEROSTOMY

he first transureteroureterostomy (TUU) in a hu-
an was described by Higgins[25] in 1935. TUU is
erformed by mobilizing the donor ureter proxi-
ally, ensuring preservation of the periureteral
dventitia. A retroperitoneal tunnel is created
cross the midline anterior to the great vessels.
lacement of the tunnel cephalad to the inferior
esenteric artery may avoid kinking depending
n the length of donor ureter available.[18,26] Mobi-
zation of the recipient ureter is minimized and a
.5-cm to 2-cm medial longitudinal ureterotomy
 made.[13] In cases involving a short donor ureter,
e recipient ureter may be further mobilized to-
/ard the midline as necessary.[27] The donor ureter
 spatulated and the anastomosis is performed
/ith interrupted or running 4-0 or 5-0 absorbable
utures over a stent placed from the donor kidney
› the recipient ureter (**Fig. 1**). Some investigators
uggest that stent placement into both ureters
educes the risk of stenosis and leakage.[28]

The length and location of a proximal ureteral
tricture determine the feasibility of TUU (ie, the
bility for the donor ureter to reach across the retro-
eritoneum).[29] For this reason, TUU may be a useful
ption for patients with a proximal ureteral stricture
ocated near the sacral margin in the context of
 radiated, reoperative, or otherwise diseased
elvis.[30] Contraindications to TUU include history
f urothelial carcinoma, genitourinary tuberculosis,

idiopathic retroperitoneal fibrosis, and nephrolithiasis because progression and/or recurrence of the
causative condition can result in compromise of
both renal units and subsequent renal failure. A
rarely used alternative to TUU is transureteropyelos-
tomy, which has a theoretic lower risk of recipient
ureteral stricture, but with the additional risk of donor
ureteral obstruction caused by kinking as it crosses
the retroperitoneum.[13]

Iwaszko and colleagues[31] (2010) reported a series of 63 patients who underwent TUU, only 10 of
whom underwent the procedure for stricture. The
most common early complication was urinary
leakage from the anastomosis (9.5%). Of the 10
who underwent TUU for stricture, the location the
stricture was only reported in 1 patient (midureter).
The complication rate was significantly higher for
patients undergoing TUU for malignancy (47.6%)
rather than benign reasons (11.9%). Of the 56 patients with follow-up imaging, patency was maintained in 96.4%. After TUU, the development of
urolithiasis was seen in 8 patients (12.7%), 3 of
whom had a previous history of urolithiasis. Six
of those patients required percutaneous nephroli-
thotomy and 1 patient underwent ureteroscopic
stone extraction.

URETEROCALICOSTOMY

Ureterocalicostomy (UC) is typically used for proximal ureteral strictures involving the ureteropelvic
junction with an intrarenal pelvis and/or scarring
of the renal hilum, thus preventing a widely patent
anastomosis between the renal pelvis and ureter
(typically seen following failure of previous pyeloplasty). Although UC is best suited for massively
hydronephrotic kidneys with thinned parenchyma,
it remains feasible with normal parenchymal thickness when a lower pole partial nephrectomy is performed to expose to the lower pole caliceal
epithelium. The ureterocalicostomy is recommended by some to be the operation of choice for
proximal ureteral obstructions in children with a
horseshoe kidney.[32] It has also proved to be a
valuable option for managing ureteral necrosis
following renal transplantation in which the native
ureter is anastomosed to the lower pole calyx.[33]
We prefer this operation for salvage of failed
robotic pyeloplasty (**Fig. 2**).

A flank incision with partial resection of the 11th
or 12th rib provides excellent exposure for the
retroperitoneal approach to UC. The kidney is
completely mobilized and the hilum is exposed.
The strictured portion of the ureteropelvic junction
and proximal ureter is excised. The renal pelvis is
closed with 4-0 absorbable sutures at the level of
the renal sinus. The lower pole of the kidney is

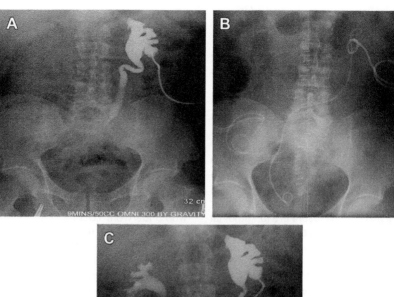

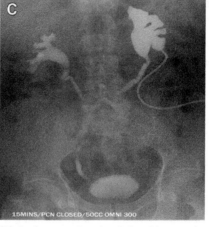

Fig. 1. Transureteroureterostomy. (*A*) Pyelogram showing left midureteral stricture. (*B*) Postoperative kidney ureter-bladder with stent spanning from donor to recipient ureter. (*C*) Pyelogram after successful TUU.

widely amputated. The desire to preserve renal parenchyma by tunneling into the lower pole should be avoided because of the increased risk of stricture with this technique.[34] Preservation of a flap of renal capsule during the amputation process may allow closure of the capsule following the anastomosis, but this is not necessary and has been postulated to increase the risk of postoperative anastomotic stricture.[24,35–37]

The renal artery may be clamped to minimize bleeding and improve visibility during anastomotic suture placement. As an alternative, local ischemia with a Penrose drain secured around the lower pole, suture ligation of the parenchymal surface, and/or argon beam coagulation may be used to limit global renal ischemia and the potential for renal artery thrombosis.[34]

After amputation of the lower pole, the spatulated ureter is sutured to the lower pole calyx using 5-0 absorbable interrupted sutures. If anastomotic tension is present, downward nephropexy from the inferior aspect of the kidney to the psoas muscle or quadratus lumborum with 2-0 nonabsorbable

suture can be performed.[24,31,38] Technical nuance of UC include vesicocalicostomy using a Boari fla and ileocalicostomy using an ileal ureter.[39,40]

Only a few large series of UC exist in the literature Osman and colleagues[36] (2011) reported a cas series of 22 patients who underwent UC. The inves tigators reported complete cure in 12 patients improvement in 4, no change in 2, and failure in 4 Of the patients who failed, 2 underwent nephrec tomy and 2 were managed with chronic double-ureteral stents. One injury to the inferior vena cav and 1 colonic injury occurred among the 22 patients Matlaga and colleagues[35] (2005) reported a serie of 11 patients who underwent UC for stricture measuring 0.5 to 3 cm with a mean follow-up o 10.1 months (range 5–32 months). None of thes patients showed recurrent obstruction as measure by intravenous urography or nuclear renography.

BLADDER FLAPS

Described by Van Hook[41] in 1893 with huma cadavers, Boari[42] with canines in 1894, and wit

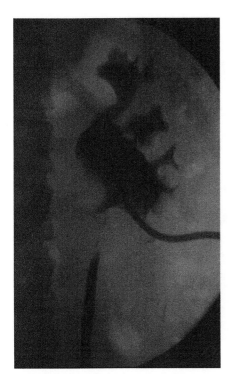

Fig. 2. Ureterocalicostomy. After 2 failed attempts with robotic pyeloplasty, this proximal ureteral stricture required ureterocalicostomy.

humans by Baidin[43] in 1930 and Ockerblad[44] in 1947, the use of bladder flaps continues to be an effective technique for complex ureteral reconstruction.[45] Although most investigators describe the Boari bladder flap (BBF) for mid ureteral strictures, Mauck and colleagues[17] (2011) showed equivalent patency rates between BBF cases performed for ureteral strictures above and below the cephalad border of the sacroiliac joint. Thus, in well-selected patients, long Boari flaps can be created that reach high into the abdomen enabling near panureteral reconstruction.

The potential length of the BBF is directly related to the patient's preoperative bladder capacity, which can be assessed with cystometrogram, cystoscopy, voiding diary, and/or retrograde cystography.[46] Although some investigators suggest that a minimum bladder capacity of 400 mL is required for BBF, other reports suggest a minimum of only 150 mL.[47,48] However, no studies have objectively measured preoperative and postoperative subjective and objective bladder function following BBF.

The BBF is performed by first releasing the bladder from its anterior attachments to the abdominal wall (obliterated umbilical arteries and urachus) and posteriorly from the peritoneum. Ligation and division of the contralateral superior vesical pedicle provides improved mobility, but great care should be taken to avoid injury to the contralateral ureter.[18,49,50] Ligation of the ipsilateral superior vesical pedicle risks compromise of the blood supply to the flap and should be avoided.

After bladder mobilization, the healthy ureter proximal to the stricture is mobilized and transected at the level of the stricture. The resulting ureteral defect is measured and an appropriately sized inverted U–shaped anterior cystotomy is made between stay sutures corresponding with the length of the defect. The length/width ratio of the bladder flap should be no more than 3:1 to preserve the vascular supply to the apex of the flap, and the base of the flap should be no less than 4 cm for the same reason.[17,48,51] A spiral orientation provides additional length for small bladders or long flaps.[52] Further length can be obtained by performing an adjunctive psoas hitch in a stepladder fashion between the flap and the psoas muscle or by making several transverse relaxing incisions on the flap.[9,53,54] The tip of the flap is then anastomosed in a refluxing fashion to the healthy end of the ureter and the flap is tubularized over a stent in a running fashion with fine absorbable suture. The tubularization continues distally until the cystotomy is completely closed (**Fig. 3**). A suprapubic tube is unnecessary unless the cystotomy closure is tenuous.

Complications seen after a BBF may include recurrent stricture, seroma, ileus, bowel obstruction, urinary tract infection, urinary leak, bladder diverticulum, and irritative voiding symptoms.[17,55] Success with the BBF is reported at greater than 90%.[17,56]

DOWNWARD NEPHROPEXY

Laparoscopic or open downward nephropexy is sometimes necessary to relieve tension on the anastomosis following ureteral reconstruction. For proximal ureteral reconstruction, the downward nephropexy is often used in conjunction with other techniques to achieve an additional 4 to 10 cm of ureteral length, thus decreasing the need for bowel interposition and its attendant risks.[17,57,58]

Downward nephropexy is performed by completely mobilizing the kidney from its attachments within the Gerota fascia. The division of the inferior adrenal artery or the left adrenal vein may also be performed, thus leaving the hilar vessels as the only remaining attachments and allowing the kidney to descend caudally.[57] The more caudal location is secured by suturing the renal capsule to either the quadratus lumborum or the psoas major muscle.

BOWEL INTERPOSITION GRAFTS

When proximal ureteral reconstruction using the native tissue is not feasible, tissue transfer

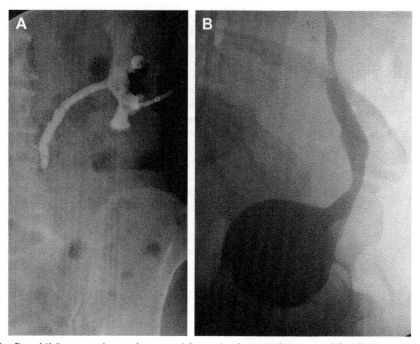

Fig. 3. Bladder flap. (*A*) Preoperative pyelogram with proximal ureteral stricture. (*B*) Following BBF, pyelography shows a widely patent reconstruction.

techniques are needed to restore ureteral continuity. Ileal ureter replacement is the preferred method for panureteral or long proximal segmental reconstruction. Additional indications for ileal ureter include a fibrotic, irradiated, and/or low-capacity bladder, which precludes safe construction of a BBF. For patients with severely decreased bladder compliance and/or capacity, an ileal ureter can be combined with bladder augmentation. Ileal ureter is also an option for bilateral ureteral substitution, allowing both renal units to drain through a single ileal segment into the bladder. Contraindications to ileal ureter include azotemia, hepatic dysfunction, inadequate length of usable bowel, untreated bladder outlet obstruction, and inflammatory bowel disease.[59,60] Although abdominopelvic radiation is not a contraindication to ileal ureter, increased complication rates can be expected in radiated patients.[61]

The technique for performing an ileal ureter echoes that of the more commonly performed ileal conduit. After mobilizing the diseased ureter and dividing it at the proximal healthy end, the length of the ureteral defect is measured and an appropriate length of distal ileum is harvested 15 cm proximal to the ileocecal valve. Bowel continuity is restored and a window is created through the colonic mesentery to position the proximal anastomosis in the retroperitoneum.[62] A refluxing end-to-end or end-to-side ureteroileal anastomosis has the lowest risk of stricture with little

risk for long-term renal damage when the ileal segment is oriented in an isoperistaltic position. A direct distal ileovesical anastomosis is also safe, simple, and imparts little risk for subsequent renal damage provided good bladder emptying is ensured (**Fig. 4**).[63]

Contemporary series of ileal ureter substitution have shown excellent results with appropriately selected patients. Matlaga and colleagues[6] (2003) published a series of 18 ileal ureter substitutions in 16 adults (preoperative creatinine 0.5–2 mg/dL) with a mean follow-up of 18.6 months that revealed no evidence of postoperative metabolic sequelae, renal insufficiency, or obstruction. Chung and colleagues[59] (2006) reported on 56 patients with 52 ileal ureters using an open refluxing ileovesical anastomosis with a mean follow-up of 6 years. Chronic kidney disease was observed in 3 patients who had preoperative azotemia. The largest series was published by Armatys and colleagues[61] (2009) with 91 patients undergoing ileal ureter substitution (99 renal units) with a mean follow-up of 36 months. Anastomotic stricture occurred in 3.3% and fistula formation in 6.6%.

The ileal ureter may be complicated by bowel obstruction, mucus obstruction, stricture (ureter, ileal graft, or anastomosis), sepsis, secondary malignancy, hernias, deep venous thrombosis, pyelonephritis, recurrent urolithiasis, wound dehiscence, chronic kidney disease, severe dilatation of the ileal limb, and metabolic acidosis.[59,64] Electrolytes

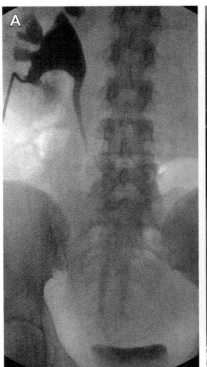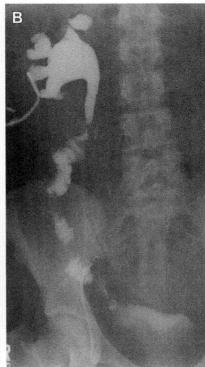

g. 4. Ileal ureter. (*A*) Preoperative pyelogram with proximal right ureteral stricture. (*B*) Antegrade pyelouretero-
ram following right ileal ureteral replacement.

hould be assessed at least annually and any meta-
olic abnormalities treated. Mucus production may
e managed with saline bladder irrigation or nightly
travesical acetylcysteine.[65] A small risk (0.8%) of
econdary malignancy exists with placement of
eum into the urinary tract with a mean latency
eriod of 18.5 years (range 12–32 years).[66,67]

Melnikoff[68] reported the first ureteral substitu-
on with appendix in 1912. The appendix is argu-
bly an ideal bowel segment for ureteral
eplacement given its caliber, which is comparable
/ith the ureter. However, the finite length of the
ppendix limits its use. Although most reports of
reteral substitution with the appendix have
ivolved the right ureter, the left ureter has also
een replaced. With normal peristalsis occurring
rom the appendiceal tip to the base, the appendix
nay be used in either isoperistaltic or antiperistal-
c direction for ureteral replacement.[69,70]

ECONFIGURED BOWEL INTERPOSITION
GRAFTS

he use of reconfigured bowel to create a urinary
onduit was described by Yang[71] (1993) and shown
n dogs by Monti and colleagues[72] (1997).
Compared with conventional ileal interposition, the
enefits of reconfigured bowel segments include a

shorter length of bowel harvested, a smaller intestinal absorptive surface, and decreased mucus
production. Both ileum and colon have been reconfigured and used as ureteral replacements in adults
and children.[69,73,74] However, the colon provides
more length when detubularized compared with
ileum because of its greater luminal diameter.
Furthermore, the colon is conveniently located in
the retroperitoneum near the ureter and away from
the bony pelvis, and thus is unaffected by any previous pelvic radiation. This close proximity of the
colon to the ureter allows for preservation of the
marginal artery when harvesting the colonic
segment. Indications for the use of colon in ureteral
replacement include dense intraperitoneal adhesions or a shortage of usable ileum.

In this technique, a 3-cm to 4-cm segment of
bowel is isolated, detubularized, and retubularized
perpendicular to its original axis to form a long
slender graft. Detubularization can be performed
in either an antimesenteric or paramesenteric
location. The latter provides an extended length
of tubularized bowel with no mesenteric attach-
ment, thus simplifying the creation of a submuco-
sal antirefluxing anastomosis with the bladder.
However, antimesenteric splitting optimizes blood
supply to each end.[75] The detubularized graft is
retubularized by closing it longitudinally over a

stent with a running 5-0 absorbable suture. The running suture is stopped before reaching the end of the tube, thus allowing a spatulated anastomosis. When the ureteral defect is too long for 1 reconfigured bowel segment, 2 segments may be used in tandem. Reconfigured colon is able to span a length of 8 to 10 cm for a single segment and 12 to 18 cm for a double segment. Although initial results with reconfigured bowel for ureteral reconstruction have been promising, larger studies with long-term follow-up are needed.[73–77]

RENAL AUTOTRANSPLANTATION

Renal autotransplantation is rarely required for complex ureteral strictures and should be used only when the previously discussed repairs are not possible or are contraindicated. Although initial reports indicated a high rate of perioperative renal loss, more contemporary series report excellent results from skilled renal transplant teams.[10,78–82]

During the nephrectomy stage of renal autotransplantation, the length of the renal artery and vein should be maximized. Immediately following nephrectomy, the kidney is flushed with an ice-cold electrolyte solution and placed in ice slush for back bench preparation. If a laparoscopic donor nephrectomy is performed, a Gibson incision may be used for both the kidney extraction and the autotransplantation.[83,84] The kidney is typically placed into the contralateral iliac fossa to maintain the vascular orientation, but this position may compromise the contralateral ureter.[85] For patients with a severely scarred renal pelvis and proximal ureteral stricture, autotransplantation may be combined with ureterocalicostomy (upper or lower pole) using the distally patent native ureter.[86]

For patients with a history of nephrolithiasis, the use of a modified pyelovesicostomy may be advisable, in which the proximal ureter is split along its posterior aspect, including the ureteropelvic junction, to create at least a 2-cm opening in the renal pelvis.[87] A bladder flap is then created using a U-shaped incision with the base of the flap at least 4 to 5 cm wide. The bladder flap is laid on the split ureter and renal pelvis, effectively creating a large spatulation of both anastomotic ends. This large spatulation may decrease the risk of anastomotic stricture and allow future stone passage, thus limiting the need for renal/ureteral endoscopy.

NEPHRECTOMY

Nephrectomy is a viable, definitive treatment option for patients with complex proximal ureteral strictures in the presence of a healthy contralateral renal unit. It is best suited for patients with lor proximal or panureteral strictures who are unfit unwilling to undergo one of the complex proce dures listed earlier or for patients with severe compromised ipsilateral renal function (<20% d ferential function).

FUTURE DIRECTIONS

Drawing on the excellent results obtained with or mucosal graft urethroplasty, several case series oral mucosal graft ureteroplasty have been re ported.[88–90] The oral mucosal grafts may b used with either an onlay or tubular techniqu commonly with incorporation of an omental wrap ping to support the graft.[91] These preliminary re ports show the feasibility of this technique, bu larger studies are needed.

Although numerous attempts have been mad to identify the ideal material for ureteral substitu tion (Box 3), most modern efforts have focuse on biologic materials. When engineering a syr thetic biologic material for ureteral replacemen a tubular acellular scaffold is often created mimic the extracellular matrix. Seeding thi

---

Box 3
Materials studied for ureteral replacement

Poly (L)-lactic acid

Autologous external jugular vein

Dermal fibroblast tubes

Human amniotic membrane

Freeze-dried arteries

Bovine dermis

Allogenic human dura mater

Porcine small intestine submucosa

Silicone-polytetrafluoroethylene–bonded tube

Polytetrafluoroethylene tube

Omentocutaneous tubularized flaps

Tubularized grafts of bladder mucosa

Tubularized collagen sponge

Polyvinyl tube

Silicone tube

Dacron tube

Self-pumping synthetic ureteral prosthesis

Dimethylpolysiloxane with polyethylene glycol terephthalate

Partial-thickness tubularized skin graft

Fallopian tube

caffold with urothelial and smooth muscle cells before surgical implantation has yielded tissues resembling normal urothelium and smooth muscle of the native ureter.[92] The results of ureteral replacement with synthetic biologic materials are promising and further research is necessary before mainstream application of these methods. Even with advances in tissue engineering, the integral principles for reconstruction of a proximal ureteral stricture remain the same.

REFERENCES

1. Assimos DG, Patterson LC, Taylor CL. Changing incidence and etiology of iatrogenic ureteral injuries. J Urol 1994;152(6 Pt 2):2240–6.
2. Siram SM, Gerald SZ, Greene WR, et al. Ureteral trauma: patterns and mechanisms of injury of an uncommon condition. Am J Surg 2010;199(4):566–70.
3. Best CD, Petrone P, Buscarini M, et al. Traumatic ureteral injuries: a single institution experience validating the American Association for the Surgery of Trauma-Organ Injury Scale grading scale. J Urol 2005;173(4):1202–5.
4. Elliott SP, McAninch JW. Ureteral injuries from external violence: the 25-year experience at San Francisco General Hospital. J Urol 2003;170(4 Pt 1):1213–6.
5. Coburn M. Damage control for urologic injuries. Surg Clin North Am 1997;77(4):821–34.
6. Stief CG, Jonas U, Petry KU, et al. Ureteric reconstruction. BJU Int 2003;91(2):138–42.
7. Austin JC. Approaches to reconstruction of the ureter. J Urol 2010;184(3):825–6.
8. Brandes S, Coburn M, Armenakas N, et al. Diagnosis and management of ureteric injury: an evidence-based analysis. BJU Int 2004;94(3):277–89.
9. Passerini-Glazel G, Meneghini A, Aragona F, et al. Technical options in complex ureteral lesions: 'ureter-sparing' surgery. Eur Urol 1994;25(4):273–80.
10. Hensle TW, Burbige KA, Levin RK. Management of the short ureter in urinary tract reconstruction. J Urol 1987;137(4):707–11.
11. Tanagho EA. A case against incorporation of bowel segments into the closed urinary system. J Urol 1975;113(6):796–802.
12. Png JC, Chapple CR. Principles of ureteric reconstruction. Curr Opin Urol 2000;10(3):207–12.
13. Armenakas NA. Current methods of diagnosis and management of ureteral injuries. World J Urol 1999;17(2):78–83.
14. Zinman LM, Libertino JA, Roth RA. Management of operative ureteral injury. Urology 1978;12(3):290–303.
15. Ubrig B, Waldner M, Roth S. Reconstruction of ureter with transverse retubularized colon segments. J Urol 2001;166(3):973–6.
16. Richter F, Stock JA, Hanna MK. The appendix as right ureteral substitute in children. J Urol 2000;163(6):1908–12.
17. Mauck RJ, Hudak SJ, Terlecki RP, et al. Central role of Boari bladder flap and downward nephropexy in upper ureteral reconstruction. J Urol 2011;186(4):1345–9.
18. Brandes SB, McAninch JW. Reconstructive surgery for trauma of the upper urinary tract. Urol Clin North Am 1999;26(1):183–99, x.
19. Bovee J. Uretero-ureteral anastomosis. Ann Surg 1897;25(1):51–79.
20. Cass AS, Schmaelzle JF, Hinman F Jr. Ureteral anastomosis in the dog comparing continuous sutures with interrupted sutures. Invest Urol 1968;6(1):94–7.
21. Tsivian A. Reconstruction of extensive upper ureteral damage. J Urol 2004;171(1):329–30.
22. Ihse I, Arnesjo B, Jonsson G. Surgical injuries of the ureter. A review of 42 cases. Scand J Urol Nephrol 1975;9(1):39–44.
23. Fry DE, Milholen L, Harbrecht PJ. Iatrogenic ureteral injury. Options in management. Arch Surg 1983;118(4):454–7.
24. Smith AD. Management of iatrogenic ureteral strictures after urological procedures. J Urol 1988;140(6):1372–4.
25. Higgins CC. Transuretero-ureteral anastomosis. J Urol 1935;34(5):349–55.
26. Borhan A, Kogan BA, Mandell J. Upper ureteral reconstructive surgery. Urol Clin North Am 1999;26(1):175–81, x.
27. Noble IG, Lee KT, Mundy AR. Transuretero-ureterostomy: a review of 253 cases. Br J Urol 1997;79(1):20–3.
28. Richter S, Kollmar O, Lindemann W, et al. Transureteroureterostomy allows renal sparing radical resection of advanced malignancies with rectosigmoid invasion. Int J Colorectal Dis 2007;22(8):949–53.
29. Sugarbaker PH, Gutman M, Verghese M. Transureteroureterostomy: an adjunct to the management of advanced primary and recurrent pelvic malignancy. Int J Colorectal Dis 2003;18(1):40–4.
30. Kamat N. Ureteric reconstruction. BJU Int 2004;93(4):635–6.
31. Iwaszko MR, Krambeck AE, Chow GK, et al. Transureteroureterostomy revisited: long-term surgical outcomes. J Urol 2010;183(3):1055–9.
32. Mollard P, Braun P. Primary ureterocalycostomy for severe hydronephrosis in children. J Pediatr Surg 1980;15(1):87–91.
33. Thevendran G, Al-Akraa MA, Sweny P, et al. Calycoureterostomy: a novel technique for post-renal transplant stricture. Surgeon 2004;2(3):176–8.

34. Ross JH, Streem SB, Novick AC, et al. Ureterocalicostomy for reconstruction of complicated pelviureteric junction obstruction. Br J Urol 1990; 65(4):322–5.

35. Matlaga BR, Shah OD, Singh D, et al. Ureterocalicostomy: a contemporary experience. Urology 2005;65(1):42–4.

36. Osman T, Eltahawy I, Fawaz K, et al. Ureterocalicostomy for treatment of complex cases of ureteropelvic junction obstruction in adults. Urology 2011; 78(1):202–7.

37. McQuitty DA, Boone TB, Preminger GM. Lower pole calicostomy for the management of iatrogenic ureteropelvic junction obstruction. J Urol 1995; 153(1):142–5.

38. Selli C, Carini M, Turini D, et al. Experience with ureterocalyceal anastomosis. Urology 1982;20(1):7–12.

39. Mandal AK, Hemal AK, Vaidyanathan S. Boari flap calycovesicostomy: a salvage procedure for giant hydronephrosis due to ureteropelvic junction obstruction. J Postgrad Med 1990;36(1):38–40.

40. Kumar A, Sharma SK, Madhusoodanan P, et al. Indications for Boari flap calicovesicostomy. Br J Urol 1988;61(4):367–8.

41. Van Hook W. The surgery of the ureters: a clinical, literary and experimental research. JAMA 1893; XXI(26):965.

42. Boari A, Casati E. Contributo sperimentale alla plastica dell'urretere. [A contribution to the experimental plastic surgery of the ureter]. Atti Accad Sci Med Nat Ferrar 1894;68:149.

43. Baidin A. The Demel autoplasty of the ureter with aid of bladder in man. Zentralbl Gynakol 1930;54: 3237–9.

44. Ockerblad NF. Reimplantation of the ureter into the bladder by a flap method. J Urol 1947;57(5):845–7.

45. Graziano M. The story of the Boari flap. J Urol 2008; 179(Suppl 4):309.

46. Chang SS, Koch MO. The use of an extended spiral bladder flap for treatment of upper ureteral loss. J Urol 1996;156(6):1981–3.

47. Kromann B, Steven K, Hald T, et al. The use of the Boari-flap and psoas-bladder hitch technique in the repair of a high ureteric lesion. A case report. Scand J Urol Nephrol 1986;20(3):233–4.

48. Stolze KJ. Boari plastic operation and reflux. Int Urol Nephrol 1972;4(1):21–4.

49. Olsson CA, Norlen LJ. Combined Boari bladder flap-psoas bladder hitch procedure in ureteral replacement. Scand J Urol Nephrol 1986;20(4): 279–84.

50. Bowsher WG, Shah PJ, Costello AJ, et al. A critical appraisal of the Boari flap. Br J Urol 1982;54(6): 682–5.

51. Hamm FC, Peng B, Waterhouse K. Experimental studies on repair of injured ureter. Arch Surg 1965;90:298–305.

52. Thompson IM, Ross G Jr. Long-term results of bladder flap repair of ureteral injuries. J Urol 1974;111(4):483–7.

53. Bhattacharya S, Overton S, Yang R, et al. Repair of upper ureteric obstruction with Boari flap and psoas hitch. Urology 1986;27(5):451–3.

54. Chary KS, Rao MS, Palaniswamy R. Vesicopyelostomy using a tubed bladder flap-multiple psoas hitch technique to an orthotopic kidney. J Urol 1982;127(1):129–31.

55. Berzeg S, Baumgart E, Beyersdorff D, et al. Late complication of Boari bladder flap. Eur Radiol 2003;13(7):1604–7.

56. Motiwala HG, Shah SA, Patel SM. Ureteric substitution with Boari bladder flap. Br J Urol 1990;66(4): 369–71.

57. Harada N, Tanimura M, Fukuyama K, et al. Surgical management of a long ureteral defect: advancement of the ureter by descent of the kidney. J Urol 1964;92:192–6.

58. Sutherland DE, Williams SB, Jarrett TW. Laparoscopic renal descensus for upper tract reconstruction. J Endourol 2011;25(2):271–2.

59. Chung BI, Hamawy KJ, Zinman LN, et al. The use of bowel for ureteral replacement for complex ureteral reconstruction: long-term results. J Urol 2006; 175(1):179–83 [discussion: 183–4].

60. Bejany DE, Lockhart JL, Politano VA. Ileal segment for ureteral substitution or for improvement of ureteral function. J Urol 1991;146(2):302–5.

61. Armatys SA, Mellon MJ, Beck SD, et al. Use of ileum as ureteral replacement in urological reconstruction. J Urol 2009;181(1):177–81.

62. Matlaga BR, Shah OD, Hart LJ, et al. Ileal ureter substitution: a contemporary series. Urology 2003;62(6):998–1001.

63. Kato H, Abol-Enein H, Igawa Y, et al. A case of ileal ureter with proximal antireflux system. Int J Urol 1999;6(6):320–3.

64. Nabizadeh I, Reid RE, Henderson JL. Simplified nonrefluxing ileovesical anastomosis. Experimental study and clinical application. Urology 1981;18(1):11–4.

65. Jang TL, Matschke HM, Rubenstein JN, et al. Pyeloureterostomy with interposition of the appendix. J Urol 2002;168(5):2106–7.

66. Austen M, Kalble T. Secondary malignancies in different forms of urinary diversion using isolated gut. J Urol 2004;172(3):831–8.

67. Ali-El-Dein B, El-Tabey N, Abdel-Latif M, et al. Late uro-ileal cancer after incorporation of ileum into the urinary tract. J Urol 2002;167(1):84–8.

68. Melnikoff AE. Sur le replacement de l'uretere par anse isolée de l'intestin grêle. Rev Clin Urol 1912; 1:601–5.

69. Obaidah A, Mane SB, Dhende NP, et al. Our experience of ureteral substitution in pediatric age group. Urology 2010;75(6):1476–80.

70. Estevao-Costa J. Autotransplantation of the vermiform appendix for ureteral substitution. J Pediatr Surg 1999;34(10):1521–3.

71. Yang WH. Yang needle tunneling technique in creating antireflux and continent mechanisms. J Urol 1993;150(3):830–4.

72. Monti PR, Lara RC, Dutra MA, et al. New techniques for construction of efferent conduits based on the Mitrofanoff principle. Urology 1997;49(1):112–5.

73. Steffens JA, Anheuser P, Reisch B, et al. Ureteric reconstruction with reconfigured ileal segments according to Yang-Monti. A 4-year prospective report. Urologe A 2010;49(2):262–7 [in German].

74. Castellan M, Gosalbez R. Ureteral replacement using the Yang-Monti principle: long-term follow-up. Urology 2006;67(3):476–9.

75. Lazica DA, Ubrig B, Brandt AS, et al. Ureteral substitution with reconfigured colon: long-term followup. J Urol 2012;187(2):542–8.

76. Ali-el-Dein B, Ghoneim MA. Bridging long ureteral defects using the Yang-Monti principle. J Urol 2003;169(3):1074–7.

77. Ubrig B, Roth S. Reconfigured colon segments as a ureteral substitute. World J Urol 2003;21(3):119–22.

78. Novick AC, Jackson CL, Straffon RA. The role of renal autotransplantation in complex urological reconstruction. J Urol 1990;143(3):452–7.

79. Webster JC, Lemoine J, Seigne J, et al. Renal autotransplantation for managing a short upper ureter or after ex vivo complex renovascular reconstruction. BJU Int 2005;96(6):871–4.

80. Lutter I, Molcan T, Pechan J, et al. Renal autotransplantation in irreversible ureteral injury. Bratisl Lek Listy 2002;103(11):437–9.

81. Wotkowicz C, Libertino JA. Renal autotransplantation. BJU Int 2004;93(3):253–7.

82. Radomski JS, Jarrell BE, Carabasi RA, et al. Renal autotransplantation and extracorporeal reconstruction for complicated benign and malignant diseases of the urinary tract. J Cardiovasc Surg 1987;28(4):413–9.

83. Meng MV, Freise CE, Stoller ML. Expanded experience with laparoscopic nephrectomy and autotransplantation for severe ureteral injury. J Urol 2003;169(4):1363–7.

84. Fabrizio MD, Kavoussi LR, Jackman S, et al. Laparoscopic nephrectomy for autotransplantation. Urology 2000;55(1):145.

85. Marshall VF, Whitsell J, McGovern JH, et al. The practicality of renal autotransplantation in humans. JAMA 1966;196(13):1154–6.

86. Greene KL, Meng MV, Abrahams HM, et al. Laparoscopic-assisted upper pole ureterocalicostomy using renal inversion and autotransplantation. Urology 2004;63(6):1182–4.

87. Flechner SM, Noble M, Tiong HY, et al. Renal autotransplantation and modified pyelovesicostomy for intractable metabolic stone disease. J Urol 2011;186(5):1910–5.

88. Sadhu S, Pandit K, Roy MK, et al. Buccal mucosa ureteroplasty for the treatment of complex ureteric injury. Indian J Surg 2011;73(1):71–2.

89. Kroepfl D, Loewen H, Klevecka V, et al. Treatment of long ureteric strictures with buccal mucosal grafts. BJU Int 2010;105(10):1452–5.

90. Badawy AA, Abolyosr A, Saleem MD, et al. Buccal mucosa graft for ureteral stricture substitution: initial experience. Urology 2010;76(4):971–5 [discussion: 975].

91. Gomez-Avraham I, Nguyen T, Drach GW. Ileal patch ureteroplasty for repair of ureteral strictures: clinical application and results in 4 patients. J Urol 1994;152(6 Pt 1):2000–4.

92. Atala A, Vacanti JP, Peters CA, et al. Formation of urothelial structures in vivo from dissociated cells attached to biodegradable polymer scaffolds in vitro. J Urol 1992;148(2 Pt 2):658–62.

Robotic Reconstruction of Lower Ureteral Strictures

Andrew P. Windsperger, MD, David A. Duchene, MD*

KEYWORDS

- Robotic • Distal ureteral reconstruction • Reimplant • Laparoscopic

KEY POINTS

- Advancements in robot-assisted laparoscopic surgery have led to the development of minimally invasive techniques for distal ureteral reconstruction.
- Enhanced visualization and range of motion with the robotic platform improves the feasibility of laparoscopic, minimally invasive distal ureteral reconstruction.
- Adjunctive procedures including vesicopsoas hitch and Boari flap are also technically feasible through a minimally invasive approach using the robotic platform.
- Initial outcomes of robotic distal ureteral reconstruction seem safe and effective, and compare well with traditional open approaches.

INTRODUCTION

The treatment of distal ureteral defects, including benign stricture disease, fistulae, and malignancy, often requires ureteral reconstruction to restore ureteral patency and normal renal drainage. Historically, distal ureteral reconstruction has been performed via open surgical intervention after failed initial endourologic management, with success rates quoted well over 90%.[1] Minimally invasive techniques for distal ureteral reconstruction were initially described nearly 2 decades ago, with reports of the first laparoscopic ureteroureterostomy by Nezhat and colleagues[2] in 1992 and laparoscopic ureteral reimplant by Ehrlich and Gershman in 1993.[3] Since that time, technological advancements in operative laparoscopy, including use of the da Vinci robotic operating platform, has allowed urologists to expand the scope of minimally invasive treatment options for distal ureteral defects.

Laparoscopic surgical approaches offer inherent benefits compared with open options when considering factors such as blood loss, hospital stay, and postoperative cosmesis. Despite this, pelvic laparoscopy often presents significant technical difficulty, and previously was reserved for those with advanced training. Use of the da Vinci operating platform across the wide scope of urology has increased surgeon comfort with minimally invasive surgery and has provided other technical benefits including three-dimensional and magnified visualization, enhanced range of motion and dexterity, and improved ease of intracorporeal suturing. Robotic surgery seems to have its greatest benefit in procedures requiring fine operative movements, where range of motion is limited, and where visibility is impeded.

Several institutions have recently described their early experience with robotic distal ureteral reconstruction, including application of supportive techniques such as vesicopsoas hitch and Boari flap creation. In this article, these publications are reviewed and the technical aspects of distal ureteral reconstruction are described. In addition to discussion of the operative technique, it is

Disclosures: None.
Department of Urology, University of Kansas Medical Center, 3901 Rainbow Boulevard, MS-3016, Kansas City, KS 66160, USA
* Corresponding author.
E-mail address: dduchene@kumc.edu

Urol Clin N Am 40 (2013) 363–370
http://dx.doi.org/10.1016/j.ucl.2013.04.006
0094-0143/13/$ – see front matter © 2013 Elsevier Inc. All rights reserved.

imperative to review factors such as patient selection and preoperative and postoperative evaluation.

PATIENT SELECTION

Patient selection is an essential factor for successful completion of a robotic distal ureteral reconstruction. As in planning for any procedure, patient comorbidity factors should be addressed and optimized before the operation. Factors such as age, body habitus and mobility, previous surgical history, and body mass index need to be considered.

Although technically feasible, robotic ureteral reconstruction in patients with morbid obesity may present additional operative challenges not encountered in the nonobese patient. Increased abdominal girth may inhibit the full range of motion of robotic arms and instruments and limit the full extension of the instruments into the pelvis. In these situations, longer trocars and instruments may assist with successful completion of the operation. Also, great care should be taken to prevent operative positioning injuries, with special attention given to padding all pressure points and areas of bony prominence.

Patients with significant past surgical histories including multiple intra-abdominal operations or use of abdominal mesh may prove to be less optimal candidates for robotic distal ureteral reconstruction. A history of previous extensive intra-abdominal surgeries is another relative contraindication to robotic ureteral reconstruction. Significant scarring and adhesion formation may impede the development of proper anatomic surgical planes. In addition, substantial adhesion formation may inhibit the ability to establish the operative domain and prolong operative times due to excessive adhesiolysis.

PREOPERATIVE EVALUATION

The overall preoperative evaluation may vary greatly from patient to patient given the etiology of distal ureteral pathologic conditions; however, proper imaging is a mainstay in patient evaluation and operative planning. The location of the pathologic lesion, the length of the affected ureteral segment, and the extent of the defect must be defined during preoperative planning as these factors may influence the type of repair. Patients often present with basic imaging that demonstrates obstruction, including axial imaging studies such as ultrasonography or computed tomography (CT) scans. Triple-phase CT scans provide particular benefit as delayed images demonstrate

ureteral filling and associated defects or obstruction. Nuclear medicine radioisotope studies including Mag-3 Lasix renograms may be of benefit in assessing the degree of preoperative obstruction, and can also be used in postoperative follow-up to demonstrate the patency of the repair. A functional study, such as a Mag-3 renogram, also confirms adequate renal function before planning repair. Depending on the presentation, some patients may undergo initial management with ureteral stent placement or nephrostomy tube placement. Retrograde pyelography and antegrade nephrostograms, or a combination of the two (an aptly named up and down-o-gram) may also provide a dynamic view of the affected ureteral segment, and provide further information for operative planning.

Patients with a history of urothelial malignancy or when an index of suspicion for malignancy exists, should undergo endoscopic evaluation via ureteroscopy with biopsy, brush biopsy, or ureteral washing. The imaging studies mentioned earlier, particularly a triple-phase contrast CT scan, generally provide sufficient information to determine whether preoperative ureteroscopy is necessary before repair.

In assessing the diseased ureteral segment, determination of the length of the potential defect to be bridged is paramount to planning the necessary repair and assisting in preoperative counseling. Defects of 2 to 3 cm may be managed with ureteroureterostomy, whereas defects of 4 to 5 cm may be better managed via ureteroneocystotomy. For defects measuring 6 to 10 cm, a vesicopsoas hitch may be more appropriate. A Boari flap or bladder advancement flap may be used for longer defects measuring 12 to 15 cm in length (**Table 1**).[4–6]

OPERATIVE EVALUATION AND PROCEDURAL POSITIONING

Before proceeding to the operating room for a robotic distal ureteral repair, medical evaluation

Table 1	
Various reconstructive techniques for lengths of ureteral defects	
Technique	**Length of Ureteral Defect (cm)**
Ureteroureterostomy	2–3
Ureteroneocystostomy	4–5
Vesicopsoas hitch	6–10
Boari flap	12–15

nd clearance from a multidisciplinary team are ecommended, including the urologic primary urgical team, the anesthetic team, and any med-al consultants if specific concerns need to be ddressed. Our patients are administered a gentle reoperative bowel preparation consisting of nagnesium citrate and a clear liquid diet the day efore the procedure. Patients should also receive ppropriate perioperative antibiotic prophylaxis n accordance with current guidelines, usually onsisting of a first-generation cephalosporin or uoroquinolone depending on allergy status. equential compression devices are placed efore induction of the general anesthetic.

After induction, the patient is placed in a dorsal thotomy position with the arms tucked at their ides. Great care should be taken to keep the rms in a slightly supinated, neutral position with ppropriate padding to avoid potential median r ulnar nerve injury. An orogastric tube is placed er anesthesia for gastric decompression. Pa-ents should be secured to the operating table ia padding and tucking of arms, or using a surgi-al bean bag immobilizer. After appropriate posi-ioning, a tilt test may be performed to ensure that he patient will tolerate a steep Trendelenberg osition without anesthetic issues or change in ositioning. Proper steps should also be taken o ensure access to nephrostomy tubes if pre-ent, as injection via the nephrostomy tube or lamping may induce hydroureter, subsequently iding in ureteral identification, dissection, and ransection. In addition, removal of the nephros-omy tube in the operating room may help to pre-ent malpositioning of any ureteral stents placed luring the repair.

Some investigators advocate performing ystoscopy with retrograde placement of a ure-eral catheter with or without a wire before the bdominal portion of the operation.[7] Ureteral tenting is a necessary part of the procedure and ids in healing of the repair; our institution has avored placement of the ureteral stent via a wire assed through an assistant port with direct visu-lization of the ureteral stent placement during the epair. Depending on the nature of the stricture, etrograde stent placement may not be possible. After cystoscopy and ureteral catheter placement r before establishing pneumoperitoneum, a Foley atheter should be placed for bladder decompres-ion. In cases where an associated vaginal defect xists such as ureteral-vaginal fistula, a sponge tick or EEA sizer inserted per vagina may assist vith visualization and dissection. In cases where he distal ureteral segment is to be excised ecause of malignancy, endoscopic scoring of he mucosa surrounding the ureteral orifice has

been advocated to facilitate removal of a bladder cuff at the time of resection.[7,8]

In addition to dorsal lithotomy positioning, pa-tients are placed in a moderate to steep Trende-lenberg position to allow the abdominal contents to fall out of the operative field as much as possible. Previous publications have indicated that tilting the table upward on the affected side, or airplaning the table, may also assist with preser-ving visualization within the operative field.[9,10] The robotic surgical system is then brought toward the operative field between the patient's legs when supine or over the ipsilateral iliac crest when in a tilted position (**Fig. 1**).

ACCESS AND PORT PLACEMENT

To establish pneumoperitoneum, an umbilical stab incision is made and a Veress needle is used to ac-cess the intraperitoneal cavity. As mentioned pre-viously, gastric and bladder decompression via orogastric tube and Foley catheter, as well as careful advancement of the Veress needle should be performed to minimize risk of damage to any intra-abdominal organs or vasculature. Aspiration of the Veress needle after initial placement can rule out bowel or vascular injury and the saline drop test may be used to confirm positioning. A pneumoperitoneum of 15 mm Hg using CO_2 gas

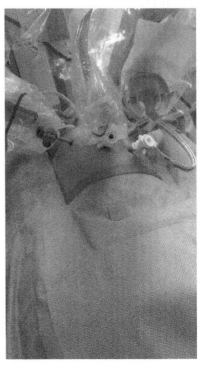

Fig. 1. Robotic console docked between patient's legs.

is established, and the umbilical insertion incision is lengthened for placement of a 12-mm camera port. The abdomen is then inspected with a 30° lens, and additional ports are placed under direct visualization; 8-mm robotic ports are placed in a triangulated position on either side of the camera port (**Fig. 2**). A 5-mm assistant port and 12-mm lateral working port may be placed either ipsilateral or contralateral to the affected side, although the authors favor placing both assistant ports contralateral to the affected side (**Fig. 3**). The robotic surgical system is docked; bipolar Maryland forceps are placed in the nondominant hand and Endoshears with monopolar cautery are placed in the dominant hand.

The initial steps of any distal ureteral reconstruction include lysis of any intra-abdominal adhesions, incision of the white line of Toldt, and medial reflection of the colon. After colonic reflection, the ureter is identified, dissected free from its surrounding attachments, and circumferential access is obtained. Great care should be taken to preserve periureteral tissue during the dissection to maximize the ureteral blood supply. The ureter may be encircled with a vessel loop (with 5-mm titanium clips on the vessel loop to secure the loop) for purposes of retraction to minimize direct trauma to the ureter.

URETEROURETEROSTOMY

Ureteroureterostomy may be an appropriate choice of reconstruction when dealing with strictures that are relatively short in length with a well-defined location. Ureteral defects of up to 2 to 3 cm may be bridged with ureteroureterostomy. After mobilization of the ureter, the diseased segment is excised and generally sent for

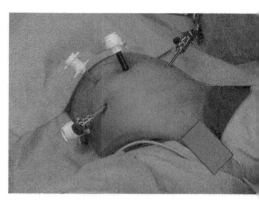

Fig. 3. Port placement for left-sided robotic distal ureteral construction.

pathologic analysis. Excision of the ureteral segment and spatulation on both ends of the ureter are performed sharply with round-tipped robotic scissors. Spatulation should be carried out at least 5 mm on both the distal and proximal ureteral segments; 4-0 polyglactin sutures are then used in either an interrupted fashion or a running fashion to complete the anastomosis. Before completion of the anastomosis, a double J stent is placed under direct visualization via the assistant port. A 0.889 mm (0.035 inch) polytetrafluoroethylene wire is advanced in the proximal ureter and the ureteral stent is guided over the wire until resistance is met. The distal end of the ureteral stent is then fed into the bladder. A peritoneal flap or omental flap may also be wrapped around the completed anastomosis to maximize the ureteral vascular supply and aid in postoperative healing.

URETERONEOCYSTOTOMY

Ureteral pathology that entails resection of the distal ureter or bridging a gap of approximately to 5 cm may be managed with ureteral neocystotomy. Once the ureter has been mobilized to the site of the affected segment or the point of distal ureteral resection, the distal end of the remaining healthy ureter is inspected and spatulated as previously described. In cases of severe stricture disease, the lumen of the affected ureteral segment is often obliterated. This segment can be managed by oversewing the ureteral stump with 4-0 polyglactin suture. After spatulating the remaining distal ureter, attention is directed toward mobilization and intraperitonealization of the bladder. The urachus is divided, and the space of Retzius is developed between the medial umbilical ligament all the way down to the endopelvic fascia. This procedure allows for a tension-free ureteral neocystotomy. When determining the site for ureteral

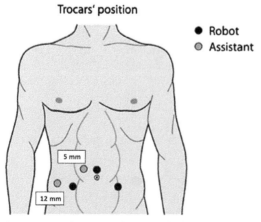

Fig. 2. Port placement for left-sided robotic distal ureteral construction.

reimplantation on the bladder, care should be taken to reimplant the ureter on the posterior aspect of the bladder and not too far anteriorly, because this may cause intermittent obstruction of the ureter with large bladder volumes. The bladder should be filled with 200 to 300 mL of saline, and the detrusor fibers should then be split to expose the underlying mucosa. Once identified, the mucosa is incised sharply to a length that matches the spatulated ureter. Our institution has favored use of 4-0 polyglactin sutures in a running fashion to achieve mucosal apposition, followed by use of intermittent 4-0 polyglactin sutures to re-approximate detrusor fibers over the neocystotomy to obtain a watertight closure and create a slight intramural tunnel. Some investigators have advocated the use of flexible cystoscopy to determine the site for reimplantation, dimming the light from the robotic camera and visualizing the light from the cystoscope to select an appropriate position on the lateral dome or posterolateral bladder wall.[9] Our institution has favored this approach in cases where excision of an associated distal ureteral lesion, such as a bladder diverticulum, must be performed.

EXTRAVESICAL URETERAL REIMPLANTATION

An extravesical ureteral reimplantation may be used in cases aimed toward correction of vesicoureteral reflux. In this procedure, the ureter itself is never transected, nor is it disassociated from its orthotopic ureteral orifice within the bladder. Ureterolysis is performed up to the beginning of the intramural tunnel. At this point, a new ureteral trough is created by filling the bladder with normal saline and incising the adjacent detrusor muscle without violation of the mucosa. After complete mobilization, the ureter is placed within this trough and the detrusor muscle is approximated over it in an interrupted fashion with 4-0 polyglactin to lengthen the intramural segment of the ureter.

URETEROVAGINAL FISTULA REPAIR

The principles of management for ureterovaginal fistulas mirror those for management of obliterative distal ureteral strictures. A direct connection may be visualized between the vaginal cuff and ureter in areas where hemostatic maneuvers were performed at the time of hysterectomy, including stapler use or suture ligation. On identification of the fistulous connection, the involved ureteral segment and fistula tract are excised and sent for pathologic analysis. With the aid of a vaginal sponge stick or EEA sizer, the vaginal defect is repaired with 2-0 polyglactin suture,

and additional interpositional grafts such as omentum or peritoneum may be used for coverage of the defect. The ureteral stump is then ligated with a suture ligation and ureter reconstructed as clinically indicated.

VESICOPSOAS HITCH

In cases where a longer ureteral defect of up to 6 to 10 cm must be bridged, a vesicopsoas hitch may be combined with ureteral reimplantation to allow for a tension-free repair. Normal bladder size and compliance aid the surgeon in performing a successful vesicopsoas hitch, and patients in whom a psoas hitch is anticipated may benefit from a preoperative evaluation of bladder capacity. After ureterolysis and transection, the bladder is intra-peritonealized and mobilized down to the level of the endopelvic fascia. The ipsilateral psoas muscle and its tendon are exposed, taking great care to identify the genitofemoral nerve as it courses over the psoas muscle. The contralateral superior bladder pedicle may be sacrificed to facilitate vesicopsoas hitch, and this may be performed using ligating clips, a vascular stapler, or vessel sealant system such as the Ligasure. Two or three 2-0 polyglactin or polydiaxonone sutures are then placed through the psoas tendon in a direction parallel to the genitofemoral nerve to avoid entrapment, and placed through the bladder to complete the vesicopsoas hitch. Ureteral reimplantation is then performed as previously described.[11,12]

BOARI FLAP AND BLADDER ADVANCEMENT FLAP

For large ureteral defects measuring 12 to 15 cm in length, a Boari flap or bladder advancement flap may be performed in addition to the vesicopsoas hitch. Initially described by Boari in a canine model in 1897, and first reported in humans in 1947, a Boari flap entails creation of an anterior bladder flap that bridges the additional ureteral gap when combined with a psoas hitch.[13] Reports of robotic Boari flap creation emerged in 2008, with additional series reported since then.[14] After transection of the ureter and mobilization of the bladder, including ligation of the contralateral superior vascular pedicle, an anterior cystotomy is created approximately 2 cm proximal to the bladder neck. The flap is carried toward the ipsilateral bladder dome, ensuring that the base of the flap remains wide enough to maintain appropriate vascular supply. Investigators have indicated that an apical flap width of 2 cm with a base flap width of 4 cm provides appropriate vascular supply.[5] The apex of the flap is then anastomosed to the distal ureter with 4-0 polyglactin suture. After ureteral anastomosis, the cystotomy is closed in a 2-layer fashion with 4-0 and 2-0 polyglactin. The flap is then gently hitched to the psoas as previously described.[15]

Alternatively, a bladder advancement flap has been proposed as an alternative to Boari flap creation. A transverse cystotomy is created at one-third of the distance between the bladder neck and ipsilateral bladder dome. The incision is extended to allow the flap to reach the distal ureter, and the apex of the flap and the ureter are then anastomosed as described for the Boari flap. The cystotomy is then closed vertically in a layered closure and the flap secured via a vesicopsoas hitch.[6]

POSTOPERATIVE CARE AND FOLLOW-UP

Patients undergo placement of closed suction drains through a designated laparoscopic port before completion of the operation: 12-mm ports are closed with 0 polyglactin sutures and use of the Carter-Thomason device; robotic and laparoscopic port sites are closed with absorbable 4-0 monofilament sutures and topical skin adhesive.

Patients are admitted for routine postoperative recovery. Subcutaneous heparin, 24-hour antibiotic prophylaxis, and a bowel regimen are initiated in addition to other care. Anticholinergics may be a useful adjunct to the postoperative pain regimen to alleviate bladder spasms or stent-related discomfort. Surgical drains are generally removed at 48 hours, or once outputs stabilize without concern for urine leak. Drain fluid may be sent for creatinine analysis to rule out evidence of postoperative urine leak. The indwelling Foley catheter is generally left in place for 5 to 10 days depending on the size of the cystotomy and quality of the repair. Ureteral stents remain in place for 4 to 6 weeks postoperatively to allow the ureteral anastomosis to heal fully.

At our institution, patients are followed on a routine basis after hospital discharge and convalescence. Nuclear medicine radioisotope MAG3 scans are obtained at 3, 9, and 18 months postoperatively to assess the patency of the repair. Patients also return for detailed symptom checks, including questionnaires to assess for bladder dysfunction after vesicopsoas hitch or Boari flap.

RESULTS AND CURRENT LITERATURE

Recent advancements in robotic surgery have led to advancements in minimally invasive urologic reconstructive techniques. These minimally invasive urologic reconstructive procedures rely on and benefit from the improved optics and three-dimensional visualization afforded by the robotic surgical operating system, as well as the improved dexterity afforded by the robotic EndoWrist's 7° of movement versus the 4° of movement offered in traditional laparoscopy. As outlined in this article, distal ureteral reconstruction is an area where advancements in robotic surgery have led to improvements in minimally invasive techniques.

In recent years, several institutions have begun to report their initial experience with robotic distal ureteral reconstruction. Until 2008, reports of robotic distal ureteral reconstructive techniques were limited to individual case reports. Robotic distal ureteral reconstruction is a relatively rare entity in urologic practice, therefore data on long-term outcomes and comparisons with alternative techniques are limited. Despite this relative paucity of literature, several of the larger published series in the recent literature are discussed here.

In 2008, Patil and colleagues[12] reported a multi-institutional review of 12 patients undergoing robotic distal ureteral reconstruction by 3 surgeons. All patients underwent a successful robotic operation with a mean operative time of 208 minutes. Average estimated blood loss was 48 mL, and at a mean follow-up of 15.5 months, all patients were clinically asymptomatic with normal renal function with a clinical success rate of 100%. Nuclear medicine radioisotope MAG3 scans demonstrated a radiographic success rate of 80% as 2 patients had minimal residual hydronephrosis. No major complications were reported.

In 2008, Schimpf and Wagner[14] reported a series of 11 patients who underwent distal ureteral reconstruction, including 3 psoas hitch procedures and 2 Boari flaps. The mean operative time in this series was 189 minutes, with a mean estimated blood loss of 82 mL. Patients all underwent successful robotic procedures and were discharged home on mean postoperative day 2.4. The investigators reported 3 major complications, including ileus, persistent hematuria requiring bladder fulguration at the neocystotomy site, and 1 intraoperative external iliac vein injury that was repaired robotically at the time of surgery. A mean follow-up of 20.5 months was reported with a clinical success rate of 82%; 2 patients reported residual postoperative flank pain despite normal radiographic findings on MAG3 scans with half-time less than 10 minutes. In 2010, Lee and colleagues[16] reported on an initial series of 3 patients who underwent robotic ureteroureterostomy. Mean operative time in this series was 136.6 minutes, and 100% clinical and radiographic success rates were reported with greater than 24 months of follow-up.

In early 2012, Baldie and colleagues[9] reported n the Emory University experience with distal robotic ureteral reconstruction compared with a cohort of patients undergoing pure laparoscopic distal ureteral reconstruction. Overall, 16 patients underwent robotic distal ureteral reconstruction: 3 reimplants and 3 ureteroureterostomies. Six patients underwent pure laparoscopic ureteral reimplantation. Two of 16 patients in the robotic group underwent conversion to open procedure, for assistance with Boari flap creation and the other for assistance with psoas hitch completion. In the laparoscopic group, 1 patient underwent conversion to open procedure to complete the ureteral anastomosis. The mean operative time was 258.6 minutes in the robotic group versus 276.5 minutes in the laparoscopic group. Mean estimated blood loss was similar at 171 mL in the robotic group and 150 mL in the laparoscopic group. Patients were discharged on mean postoperative day 2.5 in the robotic group and 2.7 in the laparoscopic group. At a mean follow-up of 8.4 months, all patients were reported to have clinical and radiographic successes. The investigators reported 3 major complications including enterotomy in 1 patient and conversion to open procedure in 2 patients.

Most recently, Kozinn and colleagues[17] reported on a series of patients from the Lahey Clinic who underwent robotic ureteral reconstruction versus a matched cohort of patients treated via open ureteral reconstruction. This series included 10 patients in the robotic group and 10 in the open group. Operative techniques included robotic neocystostomies, 4 robotic vesicopsoas hitches, and 2 robotic Boari flaps compared with neocystostomies, 3 vesicopsoas hitches, and 1 Boari flap in the open cohort. Age, gender, American Society of Anesthesiologists scores, and stricture lengths were similar between the groups. Patients in the robotic group had less blood loss than in the open group (30.6 mL vs 127.5 mL; $P = .001$), and length of stay averaged 3.4 days in the robotic group versus 5.1 days in the open group ($P = .010$). Average operative times were slightly longer in the robotic group at 306.6 minutes versus 270.0 minutes in the open group, although this difference was not statistically significant ($P = .316$). Outcomes were similar with all patients having clinical relief of obstructive symptoms and no signs of obstruction on postoperative imaging.

SUMMARY

Distal ureteral reconstruction is increasingly being. performed through minimally invasive approaches using robotic-assisted laparoscopic surgery. These studies demonstrate the safety and efficacy of robotic distal ureteral reconstruction, as well as equivalent outcomes compared with open or pure laparoscopic approaches. Additional studies will be added to the growing body of robotic literature including prospective studies for patients undergoing robotic distal ureteral reconstruction. The robotic surgical platform provides another modality for repairing distal ureteral lesions with all the associated benefits of a minimally invasive approach. Robotic distal ureteral reconstruction should be considered as a promising approach in appropriately selected patients.

REFERENCES

1. Carlton CE Jr, Guthrie AG, Scott R Jr. Surgical correction of ureteral injury. J Trauma 1969;9: 457–64.
2. Nezhat C, Nezhat F, Green B. Laparoscopic treatment of obstructed ureter due to endometriosis by resection and ureteroureterostomy: a case report. J Urol 1992;148:865–8.
3. Ehrlich RM, Gershman A. Laparoscopic seromyotomy (auto-augmentation) for non-neurogenic neurogenic bladder in a child: initial case report. Urology 1993;42:175–8.
4. Campbell MF, Wein AJ, Kavoussi LR. 10th edition. Campbell-Walsh urology, vols. 2–3. Philadelphia: Saunders Elsevier; 2011.
5. Fugita OE, Kavoussi L. Laparoscopic ureteral reimplantation for ureteral lesion secondary to transvaginal ultrasonography for oocyte retrieval. Urology 2001;58:281.
6. Lima GC, Rais-Bahrami S, Link RE, et al. Laparoscopic ureteral reimplantation: a simplified dome advancement technique. Urology 2005;66:1307.
7. Uberoi J, Harnisch B, Sethi AS, et al. Robot-assisted laparoscopic distal ureterectomy and ureteral reimplantation with psoas hitch. J Endourol 2007;21(4): 368–73 [discussion: 372–3].
8. Phillips EA, Wang DS. Current status of robot-assisted laparoscopic ureteral reimplantation and reconstruction. Curr Urol Rep 2012;13(3):190–4.
9. Baldie K, Angell J, Ogan K, et al. Robotic management of benign mid and distal ureteral strictures and comparison with laparoscopic approaches at a single institution. Urology 2012;80:596–601.
10. Muffarrij PW, Shah OD, Berger AD, et al. Robotic reconstruction of the upper urinary tract. J Urol 2007;278:2002.
11. Naeyer GD, Migem PV, Schatteman P, et al. Pure robot-assisted psoas hitch ureteral reimplantation for distal-ureteral stenosis. J Endourol 2007;21: 618–20.

12. Patil NN, Mottrie A, Sundaram B, et al. Robotic-assisted laparoscopic ureteral reimplantation with psoas hitch: a multi-institutional, multinational evaluation. Urology 2008;72:47.

13. Ockerblad NF. Reimplantation of the ureter into the bladder by a flap method. J Urol 1947;57: 845.

14. Schimpf MO, Wagner JR. Robot-assisted laparoscopic Boari flap ureteral reimplantation. J Endourol 2008;22:2691.

15. Modi P, Goel R, Dodiya S. Laparoscopic ureteroneocystostomy for distal ureteral injuries. Urology 200 66:751.

16. Lee DI, Schwab CW, Harris A. Robot-assisted ur teroureterostomy in the adult: initial clinical serie Urology 2010;75:570–3.

17. Kozinn SI, Canes D, Sorcini A, et al. Robotic versu open distal ureteral reconstruction and reimplanta tion for benign stricture disease. J Endourol 201 26(2):147–51.

Standardized Approach for the Treatment of Refractory Bladder Neck Contractures

Daniel Ramirez, MD[a], Jay Simhan, MD[a],
Steven J. Hudak, MD[b], Allen F. Morey, MD[a],*

KEYWORDS

• Bladder neck contracture • Refractory • Balloon dilation • Stricture

KEY POINTS

• BNC is associated with surgical factors during prostatectomy, smoking history, diabetes, coronary vascular disease, and pelvic radiation.
• Urethral stenting has high rate of complication and need for reoperation.
• Urethral dilation and endosopic incision are successful in the great majority of patients with BNC.
• Transurethral injection therapy is a promising option for refractory BNC.
• Open reconstruction remains a viable option for refractory BNC when endoscopic management fails.
• Management of stress urinary incontinence after BNC treatment can be safely performed after stability of bladder neck is determined.

INTRODUCTION

With the number of patients treated by radical prostatectomy (RP) or radiation for localized prostate cancer on the rise,[1] the development of bladder neck contracture (BNC; **Fig. 1**) after treatment remains a recognized complication treated by urologists in contemporary practice today.[2] Although the incidence of BNC after RP has continued to decrease over the last 20 years with the advent of robotic surgery and refinements in surgical technique, a small subset of patients nevertheless develop anastomotic strictures warranting treatment.[2–4] Many patients undergoing initial treatment of BNC achieve successful early results,[5–10] but a significant group of patients experience recurrent obstruction. As a result, patients with refractory BNC pose a difficult clinical management scenario for urologists. Although recent efforts have focused on determining factors associated with the occurrence of BNC[2,3,11–13] to better direct prevention and treatment, the management of refractory disease remains challenging and unstandardized. Most contractures are often managed successfully with conservative measures, such as serial dilation or transurethral incision, with acceptable success rates ranging from 50% to 87%.[11,12,14,15]

When conservative approaches fail, patients with refractory BNC require additional treatments with increasing procedural complexity (**Fig. 2**). As such, patients with refractory and recurrent BNC

Disclaimer: The opinions expressed in this document are solely those of the authors and do not represent an endorsement by or the views of the United States Air Force, the United States Army, the Department of Defense or the United States Government.
[a] Department of Urology, UT Southwestern Medical Center, Moss Building, 8th Floor, Suite 112, 5323 Harry Hines Boulevard, Dallas, TX 75390–9110, USA; [b] Department of Surgery, Urology Section, San Antonio Military Medical Center, 3551 Roger Brooke Drive, Fort Sam Houston, TX 78234, USA
* Corresponding author.
E-mail address: Allen.Morey@utsouthwestern.edu

Urol Clin N Am 40 (2013) 371–380
http://dx.doi.org/10.1016/j.ucl.2013.04.012
0094-0143/13/$ – see front matter © 2013 Elsevier Inc. All rights reserved.

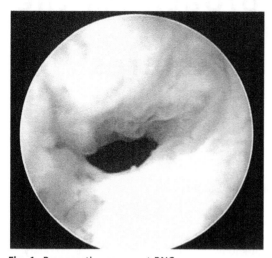

Fig. 1. Preoperative recurrent BNC.

present a challenging management dilemma that is the focus of this article. Here we summarize various methods used to manage patients with refractory BNC at our institution.

BACKGROUND: CAUSES AND INCIDENCE OF BNC WITH ASSOCIATED RISK FACTORS

The primary treatment sustained by the patient often plays a central role in the cause of BNC development. In patients undergoing pelvic radiation therapy for malignancy, microvascular effects and progressive obliterative endarteritis leading to tissue necrosis of the bladder neck is a well-described phenomenon.[16,17] Conversely, in patients undergoing RP, it is often suggested that BNC arises because of technical factors surrounding surgery. Prior reports have suggested that most BNC can be prevented during RP in particular through a tension-free watertight anastomosis

and mucosal eversion at the time of surgery. Thus, it is not surprising that the incidence of BNC has decreased after robotic-assisted laparoscopic prostatectomy (0%–3%)[2,3,18] when compared with historical data after open RP (0.5%–32%).[2,9,11,1] BNC is also a well-known complication of endoscopic treatment of benign prostatic hyperplasia. Although conventional transurethral resection of the prostate was noted to have a BNC rate between 1% and 12.3%,[20,21] a smaller rate of BNC has been noted with newer technologies, such as the KTP laser prostatectomy (3%–5%).[22–24]

Many proposed factors contribute to the development of BNC after prostate surgery, including surgical technique, surgeon experience, postoperative complications, and patient comorbidities (**Box 1**). In a retrospective analysis of 467 patients undergoing RP, Borboroglu and colleagues[1] studied the development of BNC in 52 patients. Through a multivariable analysis assessing for predictors of BNC, the authors discovered that intraoperative blood loss, increased operative time, a positive smoking history, diabetes mellitus, and the presence of coronary artery disease were all significant predictors linked to the development of BNC. In our institution, we have also noted a significant correlation between a greater than 1-pack per year smoking history and the development of recurrent BNC when compared with nonsmokers.

A recent review of the Cancer of the Prostate Strategic Urologic Research Endeavor database revealed that patient age, body mass index, and primary type of treatment were all prognostic indicators for the development of clinically significant strictures requiring treatment in patients undergoing primary treatment of localized prostate cancer.[25] This analysis also demonstrated that although BNC after prostatectomy typically

| Serial urethral dilation

Clean intermittent catheterization | Endoscopic balloon dilation with incision of bladder neck (UTSW)

Urethral stenting with UroLume (Anger et al, 2005)

Urethrotomy with injection of steroid (Eltahawy et al, 2008) or Mitomycin C (Vanni et al, 2011) | Abdominoperineal excision of bladder neck with anastomosis (Theodoros et al, 2000)

Open bladder neck reconstruction (Mundy et al, 2012)

Primary excision of bladder neck with end-to-end anastomosis, penile fasciocutaneous flap, free graft urethroplasty (Wessells et al, 1998) |

INCREASING PROCEDURAL COMPLEXITY

Fig. 2. Increasing procedural severity for the treatment of refractory BNC. Patients often proceed from conservative therapy (eg, serial urethral dilation) to more intense surgical intervention for management of recalcitrant BNC.

resents within 6 months after surgery,[25] patients treated with primary radiation often present years after treatment likely because of progressive radiation-induced fibrosis and necrosis.[26] After multimodal radiotherapy (eg, brachytherapy plus external-beam radiotherapy or salvage prostatectomy), even higher rates of BNC have been reported with devastating consequences to the bladder outlet and patient quality of life.[27,28]

URETHRAL STENT PLACEMENT

The UroLume (American Medical Systems, Minnetonka, MN) was introduced in 1988 by Milroy as a novel, minimally invasive stent to manage urethral stricture disease.[29] Although initial studies regarding the use of the UroLume were promising, numerous problems were encountered with urethral stenting, including stent migration, obstruction secondary to tissue in-growth, hematuria, stent encrustation, and the need for repeat surgery.[30–35]

Stent migration, in particular, had been reported in 23% of cases[36] and additional studies had demonstrated that the onset of stent migration manifested anywhere between 6 weeks and 3 years after initial UroLume placement.[36,37] Although a 100% success rate was noted in the eight patients initially studied by Milroy and colleagues,[29] a subsequent report by Hussain and colleagues[35] demonstrated a complication rate of 50% in 60

patients that underwent urethral stenting. De Vocht and colleagues[34] also reported concerning rates of persistent urinary incontinence (50%) and a notable proportion of patients (27%) undergoing surgical revision secondary to stent obstruction.

Although initial efforts to define the role of UroLume placement focused on the management of urethral stricture disease and detrusor-sphincter dyssynergia, a recent report by Erickson and colleagues[38] evaluated the application of the UroLume specifically in patients who had undergone primary radiation or surgery for the treatment of prostate cancer. In a series that included 38 men, the study investigators reported an initial success rate of 47% with 53% (N = 19) of patients requiring repeat intervention for stent complications. As such, because of the frequency of postprocedural complications and need for further surgical treatment, urethral stenting is now rarely indicated. At our institution, the use of the UroLume stent has been abandoned because patients with bladder outlet obstruction secondary to BNC have been managed with acceptable rates of success through endoscopic balloon dilation and incisional procedures.

URETHRAL DILATION AND ENDOSCOPIC INCISION

Initial management of patients with BNC has conventionally centered on conservative measures in lieu of invasive surgical maneuvers. Intermittent dilation of the bladder neck has therefore been used to treat contractures and prevent recurrent disease. If the lumen of the contracture is amenable to urethral catheterization, gradual dilation may be performed in a clinical setting or with the use of an outpatient serial dilation program. As such, several prior works have assessed the efficacy of urethral dilation in the management of BNC after RP. In a large series (N = 510) of postprostatectomy patients in the United Kingdom, a BNC rate of 9.4% (N = 48) occurred with all patients successfully managed through urethral dilation or clean intermittent catheterization.[39] Similarly, Park and colleagues[40] used a regimen of urethral dilation to 18F catheter followed by a 3-month period of intermittent self-catheterization in 32 postprostatectomy patients with BNC. With at least 1 year of follow-up, 93% (N = 24) of patients were successfully treated with one or two dilations followed by self-catheterization. Although self-catheterization provides a nonsurgical approach to BNC management, significant patient tolerance and compliance seem to be necessary for successful results. Additionally, some patients experience complications of self-dilation, such as the development of urinary tract infection, hematuria, false passage, and urethral stricture.

An alternative technique with low procedural morbidity involves a cold-knife endoscopic incision of the bladder neck for patients with BNC.[6,7,13,15,41–43] Although numerous studies have evaluated the efficacy of cold-knife urethrotomy in first-time diagnoses of BNC, most reports have limited patient follow-up and do not report long-term results of patients undergoing multiple endoscopic treatments for recurrent stenosis. In a large series (N = 52) of BNC undergoing intervention, 22 patients (42%) required at least one repeat dilation or transurethral incision, whereas six patients (11.5%) required more than two therapeutic interventions.[11] Thus, when repeat dilation or endoscopic therapy for recurrent BNCs is necessary, subsequent success rates are inferior to those of initial transurethral incision or dilation.

Taking into account the known risks of repeat endoscopic therapy in patients with highly refractory disease, a hybrid endoscopic procedure incorporating both balloon dilation and incision has recently been developed at our institution. A brief description of this endoscopic technique is included next.

Surgical Approach and Procedure

Instruments that should be available to the surgeon during transurethral incision of a recurrent BNC are listed in **Box 2**. A 3% sorbitol solution should be used for irrigation. The case is started with careful examination of the entire urethra with a flexible cystoscope or 21F catheter rigid cystoscope. A 0.083-in Amplantz Super Stiff Guide Wire is passed through the BNC into the bladder (**Fig. 3**). With the

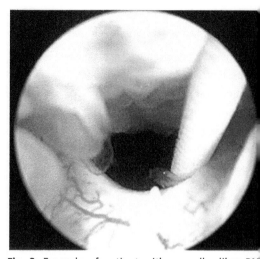

Fig. 3. Example of patient with a small-caliber BN (<6F catheter) with Super Stiff Guide wire traversin area of stenosis.

wire in place, a 4-cm, 24F catheter UroMax Ultr High Pressure dilating urethral balloon (Boston Sc entific, Natick, MA, USA) is advanced over the Su per Stiff Guide Wire (Boston Scientific, Natick, M/ USA) through the BNC. Balloon dilation of the ure thra is performed under direct vision through a 21 catheter rigid cystoscope or alongside a 16F cath eter flexible cystoscope to verify that the dilatin balloon is engaged within the contracture. Dilatio to a pressure level of 15 atm is performed with th use of the LeVeen pressure syringe (**Fig. 4**) unde direct cystoscopic vision to ensure that the balloo does not migrate during active dilation. The balloo

---

Box 2
List of instruments for endoscopic balloon dilation/transurethral incision of bladder neck contracture

Monopolar energy source

3% sorbitol irrigation solution

21F catheter rigid cystoscope

0.083-in Amplantz Super Stiff Guide wire

4-cm, 24F catheter UroMax dilating balloon

16F catheter flexible cystoscope

LeVeen pressure syringe

24F catheter resectoscope

Collings knife

22F catheter two-way soft Foley catheter

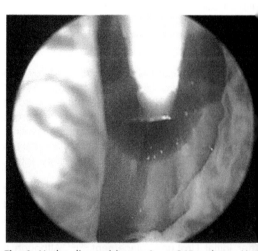

Fig. 4. Under direct vision, a 4-cm, 24F catheter Urc Max ultra high-pressure dilating urethral balloon i advanced into the bladder. Dilation to a pressure leve of 17 atm is performed using a LeVeen pressur syringe.

then left in place dilated across the area of stenosis for approximately 3 minutes to allow scar tissue
around the area of contracture to conform to a
round configuration. After this is complete, the
balloon and the wire may be removed after cystoscopy is performed to ensure no synchronous
bladder lesions or stones are present.

After the contracture has been dilated, a 24F
resectoscope is passed into the bladder using a
visual obturator. A Collings knife is attached to
the working element for use with a monopolar energy source and passed under vision into the resectoscope. Deep incisions are made at the
3-o'clock and 9-o'clock positions with a cutting
current of 30 to 50 V (**Fig. 5**). The incisions should
be carried down through the circular fibers of the
bladder neck into the perivesical fat. Injection of
antiproliferative agents, such as steroids or mitomycin C, is not required provided adequate depth
of incision is performed. After the BNC has been
incised, the lumen of the bladder neck appears
to open in a transverse fashion and the resistance
on the sides of the scope can be felt to be greatly
reduced with adequate incision depth. The scar
tissue at the posterior and anterior bladder neck
are not resected or incised. Careful hemostasis is
then obtained after evaluation under low bladder
pressures.

A 22F catheter is left in place for 5 days. Office
cystoscopy and uroflowmetry are then performed
at 2 months to assess bladder neck patency. Success in our series of patients is defined as the ability
to cannulate the bladder with a 16F catheter flexible
cystoscope in clinic (**Fig. 6**). At our institution,
patients undergoing this standardized procedure
have a success rate of 72% after one procedure,
and 86% after a single repeat balloon dilation procedure. Only 8.3% of patients required repeat
transurethral incision of recurrent contractures.
Patients with refractory BNC who fail multiple transurethral attempts at treatment should be considered for open bladder neck reconstruction by a
reconstructive specialist. **Fig. 7** summarizes the
long-term management approach of patients undergoing transurethral balloon dilation and incision
of BNC at our institution.

OPEN RECONSTRUCTION TECHNIQUES FOR BNC

Patients with long areas of contracture not
amenable to endoscopic procedures, devastating
bladder neck stenoses suffered from distraction
injuries, or those that fail numerous endoscopic
maneuvers merit consideration for open bladder
neck reconstruction. Both technically challenging

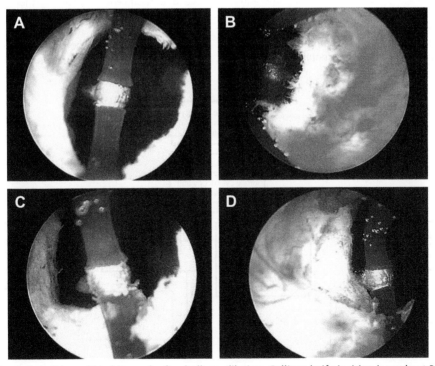

Fig. 5. Endoscopic incision of bladder neck after balloon dilation. Collings knife incision is made at 3 o'clock (*B*) and 9 o'clock (*A, C, D*). Incisions should be carried down through the circular fibers of the bladder neck into the perivesical fat (*C*).

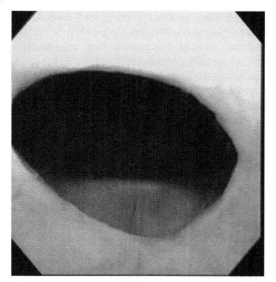

Fig. 6. Postoperative bladder neck after endoscopic therapy. This is a patent bladder neck as visualized in a patient undergoing office cystoscopy 2 months postoperatively after endoscopic balloon dilation with incision of the bladder neck.

and of greater morbidity, various approaches (abdominoperineal, perineal, and transpubic) have been reported from high-volume reconstruction centers.[44–46]

The challenging nature of these techniques mandates such procedures to be performed by experienced reconstructive surgeons with a wide-ranging treatment armamentarium. Most reports that detail operative technique for open bladder neck reconstruction are limited by small single-institutional series, short patient follow-up, or limited reproducibility of the reported findings. Nevertheless, several studies reporting on the technique and indications of open bladder neck reconstruction deserve mention.

In one of the first reports of patients with devastating bladder outlets after RP, Schlossberg and colleagues[44] described a detailed approach at abdominoperineal reconstruction of the bladder neck in two patients with prostate cancer. In their report, the investigators also described an abdominal approach combined with partial pubectomy and suggested such a technique may provide the best chance of appropriate bladder neck mobilization with preservation of urinary continence when an intact external urinary sphincter was present. Perineal approaches to BNC management have also been described in the treatment of those with refractory disease. In a case series of six patients, Simonato and colleagues[47] demonstrated acceptable results with end-to-end posterior urethroplasty and subsequent artificial urinary sphincter (AUS) placement in the management of refractory BNC. Because such approaches allow for the use of adjacent tissue transfer and for better exposure in an open fashion, the investigators suggested that perineal procedures provided for an optimal anastomotic repair in those with extensive and recurrent disease. Further defining the critical role of AUS implantation in patients undergoing open surgery, Mundy and colleagues[4] recently reported satisfactory results in 21 of 23 patients undergoing transperineal revision of the

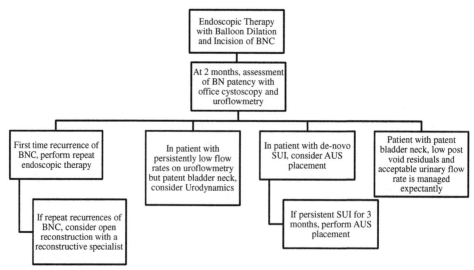

Fig. 7. Long-term management algorithm for patients undergoing endoscopic balloon dilation and incision of BNC. The following diagram summarizes the long-term approach we undertake at our institution for patients undergoing endoscopic therapy. AUS, artificial urinary sphincter; SUI, stress urinary incontinence.

esicourethral anastomosis after RP with all pa-
ents requiring subsequent AUS placement.

In select patients, a combined abdominoperi-
eal approach may be necessary for optimal visu-
ization, scar excision, tissue mobilization, or
econstruction of the bladder outlet.[45] Because
eported perineal approaches to refractory BNC
ave demonstrated the likelihood of progressive
ress urinary incontinence (SUI) secondary to
obilization and injury to the external urethral
ohincter at the time of surgery, some suggest
US implantation at the time of scar excision or
hortly thereafter.[45,47,48] Additionally, preliminary
ndings reported by Reiss and colleagues[49] re-
iewed 15 patients with recalcitrant BNC managed
y perineal bladder neck reconstruction. Reported
uccess rates after the combined approach were
igh (93%) with an acceptable patient satisfaction
ate of 93%. As such, with appropriate selection,
atient satisfaction after major perineal recon-
tructive procedures seems to have favorable
esults.

MANAGEMENT OF DE NOVO STRESS URINARY INCONTINENCE AFTER BNC TREATMENT

atients with BNC undergoing definitive endo-
copic or open surgical treatment may also
ave de novo SUI unmasked after RP at a rate
etween 2% and 7%[50–52] in high-volume series.
Ve have found the rate of de novo SUI after
UIBNC (transurethral incision of bladder neck
ontracture) in patients presenting after RP, tran-
urethral resection of the prostate, and KTP laser
rostatectomy to be only about 4%. Data seem
o be conflicting on long-term sequelae after
ransurethral incision, with several investigators
eporting significant rates of de novo SUI un-
hasked by treatment,[15,40,41] whereas others
ave noted negligible rates of incontinence after
ndoscopic manipulation.[7,10,11,42,43]

However, the management of de novo SUI with
ubsequent AUS implantation has been studied in
atients undergoing UroLume placement. In a report
mited by small sample size, Elliott and Boone[30]
valuated nine patients who underwent bladder
eck stent placement followed by AUS implantation.
Vith a mean follow-up of 17.5 months, the investiga-
ors reported only one failure secondary to recurrent
3NC. However, in a larger analysis of 40 patients
vith longer follow-up (mean, 37 months), Borawski
nd Webster[53] discovered that 50% of patients
N = 20) undergoing urethral stenting with subsequent AUS placement required a mean 2.2 addi-
ional procedures for the treatment of stent
cclusion or AUS erosion.

Furthermore, a greater proportion (25%–45%) of
patients undergoing salvage prostatectomy experience de novo SUI after management of their BNC,
necessitating AUS placement in the management
of refractory BNC.[54,55] At our institution, patients
rarely develop de novo SUI after endoscopic BNC
treatment, whereas most present at the time of evaluation with concomitant BNC and SUI.

At our institution, after endoscopic balloon dilation and incision, patients with de novo SUI are
managed expectantly for 3 months to ensure
bladder neck stability before proceeding with
AUS implantation. If they are patent at 3 months,
we have found it to be extremely rare that they
proceed to recurrent obstruction, and we then
consider them candidates for AUS placement. If
refractory BNC after endoscopic treatment with delayed AUS placement is noted, a 12F catheter Foley
catheter may be placed for several days across a
deactivated AUS cuff. Alternatively, a suprapubic
catheter may be placed to avoid placement of a
catheter across the artificial urinary cuff. Refractory
BNC after AUS placement can be safely incised using a 200-mm Holmium laser fiber though a flexible
ureteroscope, thus minimizing the risk of potential
damage to the AUS cuff. A 12F catheter is left in
place after surgery with plans for catheter removal
decided on a case by case basis. To our knowledge, no prior studies have previously assessed
cohorts of patients who have undergone this procedure in such a setting of refractory BNC. We sur-
mise that such patients are at a high risk of failure
because of the restricted ability to perform a standardized incisional procedure. If the BNC recurs
in this setting, consideration must be made at
removal of the artificial urinary cuff until the BNC
is treated and stabilized. Alternatively, open reconstruction of the bladder neck may be undertaken by
a reconstructive specialist.

EXPERIMENTAL TECHNIQUES

Although conventional approaches to refractory
BNC include endoscopic therapy through incision
or dilation or open surgical excision with reanastomosis, experimental techniques involving resection with the holmium laser or injection of
medications at the site of the BNC have recently
been reported. With 2 years of follow-up, Eltahawy
and colleagues[56] reported an 83% success rate in
BNC treatment in 24 patients undergoing holmium
laser incision followed by injection of 80 mg triam-
cinolone at the contracture site. Other authors
have reported similar success rates using deep
cold-knife radial incisions followed by an injection
of 0.4 mg of mitomycin C to prevent recurrence of
scar formation.[57]

Although these reports suggest promising results that need to be validated by other high-volume centers, concerns regarding long-term effects of such medications have been raised by recent animal studies demonstrating impaired urothelial wound healing.[58] Furthermore, recent clinical reports have indicated adverse reactions, such as perivesical necrosis in the setting of extravasation after mitomycin C treatment[59,60] or anaphylactic reactions observed after steroid injections.[61] Although the preliminary results of injection therapy are promising, further work is necessary to delineate the role and long-term effects of such treatments at the time of bladder neck incision in the management of patients with refractory BNC.

SUMMARY

The development of refractory BNC is a relatively uncommon but well-described condition observed primarily in men undergoing treatment of prostate cancer. Although the incidence of BNC has decreased in recent years, management of this condition remains challenging. Risk factors for the development of refractory BNC include a positive history of smoking, coronary artery disease, and poorly controlled diabetes mellitus. Numerous treatment options exist for this condition varying in procedural severity, including serial urethral dilation, endoscopic maneuvers, and open reconstructive techniques. For the treatment of refractory BNC a combination of endoscopic balloon dilation and transurethral incision of the bladder neck has demonstrated a high rate of first-time therapeutic success. With a known and acceptable risk of unmasking de novo SUI, our management of patients with BNC also involves close patient follow-up with the possibility for subsequent AUS placement. Although most patients experience success with our reported endoscopic technique for refractory BNC, open bladder neck reconstruction is an option that should be reserved for the highest complexity refractory cases that have failed prior minimally invasive maneuvers.

REFERENCES

1. Cooperberg MR, Moul JW, Carroll PR. The changing face of prostate cancer. J Clin Oncol 2005; 23(32):8146–51.
2. Breyer BN, Davis CB, Cowan JE, et al. Incidence of bladder neck contracture after robot-assisted laparoscopic and open radical prostatectomy. BJU Int 2010; 106(11):1734–8.
3. Msezane LP, Reynolds WS, Gofrit ON, et al. Bladder neck contracture after robot-assisted laparoscopic radical prostatectomy: evaluation of incidence and risk factors and impact on urinary function. J Endourol 2008;22(1):97–104.
4. Carlsson S, Nilsson AE, Schumacher MC, et al. Surgery-related complications in 1253 robot assisted and 485 open retropubic radical prostatectomies at the Karolinska University Hospital, Sweden. Urology 2010;75(5):1092–7.
5. Brodak M, Kosina J, Pacovsky J, et al. Bipolar transurethral resection of anastomotic strictures after radical prostatectomy. J Endourol 2010;24(9): 1477–81.
6. Carr LK, Webster GD. Endoscopic management of the obliterated anastomosis following radical prostatectomy. J Urol 1996;156(1):70–2.
7. Dalkin BL. Endoscopic evaluation and treatment of anastomotic strictures after radical retropubic prostatectomy. J Urol 1996;155(1):206–8.
8. Giannarini G, Manassero F, Mogorovich A, et al. Cold-knife incision of anastomotic strictures after radical retropubic prostatectomy with bladder neck preservation: efficacy and impact on urinary continence status. Eur Urol 2008;54(3):647–56.
9. Kostakopoulos A, Argiropoulos V, Protogerou V, et al. Vesicourethral anastomotic strictures after radical retropubic prostatectomy: the experience of a single institution. Urol Int 2004;72(1):17–20.
10. Ramchandani P, Banner MP, Berlin JW, et al. Vesicourethral anastomotic strictures after radical prostatectomy: efficacy of transurethral balloon dilation. Radiology 1994;193(2):345–9.
11. Borboroglu PG, Sands JP, Roberts JL, et al. Risk factors for vesicourethral anastomotic stricture after radical prostatectomy. Urology 2000;56(1):96–100.
12. Geary ES, Dendinger TE, Freiha FS, et al. Incontinence and vesical neck strictures following radical retropubic prostatectomy. Urology 1995; 45(6):1000–6.
13. Gillitzer R, Thomas C, Wiesner C, et al. Single center comparison of anastomotic strictures after radical perineal and radical retropubic prostatectomy. Urology 2010;76(2):417–22.
14. Mark S, Perez LM, Webster GD. Synchronous management of anastomotic contracture and stress urinary incontinence following radical prostatectomy. J Urol 1994;151(5):1202–4.
15. Surya BV, Provet J, Johanson KE, et al. Anastomotic strictures following radical prostatectomy: risk factors and management. J Urol 1990;143(4): 755–8.
16. Hall EJ, Astor M, Bedford J, et al. Basic radiobiology. Am J Clin Oncol 1988;11(3):220–52.
17. Turina M, Mulhall AM, Mahid SS, et al. Frequency and surgical management of chronic complications related to pelvic radiation. Arch Surg 2008; 143(1):46–52 [discussion: 52].
18. Gonzalgo ML, Pavlovich CP, Trock BJ, et al. Classification and trends of perioperative morbidities

following laparoscopic radical prostatectomy. J Urol 2005;174(1):135–9 [discussion: 139].

19. Davidson PJ, van den Ouden D, Schroeder FH. Radical prostatectomy: prospective assessment of mortality and morbidity. Eur Urol 1996;29(2): 168–73.

20. Lee YH, Chiu AW, Huang JK. Comprehensive study of bladder neck contracture after transurethral resection of prostate. Urology 2005;65(3):498–503 [discussion: 503].

21. Puppo P, Bertolotto F, Introini C, et al. Bipolar transurethral resection in saline (TURis): outcome and complication rates after the first 1000 cases. J Endourol 2009;23(7):1145–9.

22. Kim HS, Cho MC, Ku JH, et al. The efficacy and safety of photoselective vaporization of the prostate with a potassium-titanyl-phosphate laser for symptomatic benign prostatic hyperplasia according to prostate size: 2-year surgical outcomes. Korean J Urol 2010;51(5):330–6.

23. Malde S, Rajagopalan A, Patel N, et al. Potassium-titanyl-phosphate laser photoselective vaporization for benign prostatic hyperplasia: 5-year follow-up from a district general hospital. J Endourol 2012; 26(7):878–83.

24. Sandhu JS, Ng C, Vanderbrink BA, et al. High-power potassium-titanyl-phosphate photoselective laser vaporization of prostate for treatment of benign prostatic hyperplasia in men with large prostates. Urology 2004;64(6):1155–9.

25. Elliott SP, Meng MV, Elkin EP, et al. Incidence of urethral stricture after primary treatment for prostate cancer: data From CaPSURE. J Urol 2007;178(2):529–34 [discussion: 534].

26. Marks LB, Carroll PR, Dugan TC, et al. The response of the urinary bladder, urethra, and ureter to radiation and chemotherapy. Int J Radiat Oncol Biol Phys 1995;31(5):1257–80.

27. Moreira SG Jr, Seigne JD, Ordorica RC, et al. Devastating complications after brachytherapy in the treatment of prostate adenocarcinoma. BJU Int 2004;93(1):31–5.

28. Zelefsky MJ, Whitmore WF Jr. Long-term results of retropubic permanent 125iodine implantation of the prostate for clinically localized prostatic cancer. J Urol 1997;158(1):23–9 [discussion: 29–30].

29. Milroy EJ, Chapple CR, Cooper JE, et al. A new treatment for urethral strictures. Lancet 1988; 1(8600):1424–7.

30. Elliott DS, Boone TB. Combined stent and artificial urinary sphincter for management of severe recurrent bladder neck contracture and stress incontinence after prostatectomy: a long-term evaluation. J Urol 2001;165(2):413–5.

31. Corujo M, Badlani GH. Epithelialization of permanent stents. J Endourol 1997;11(6):477–80.

32. Beier-Holgersen R, Brasso K, Nordling J, et al. The "Wallstent": a new stent for the treatment of urethral strictures. Scand J Urol Nephrol 1993; 27(2):247–50.

33. Morgia G, Saita A, Morana F, et al. Endoprosthesis implantation in the treatment of recurrent urethral stricture: a multicenter study. Sicilian-Calabrian Urology Society. J Endourol 1999;13(8):587–90.

34. De Vocht TF, van Venrooij GE, Boon TA. Self-expanding stent insertion for urethral strictures: a 10-year follow-up. BJU Int 2003;91(7):627–30.

35. Hussain M, Greenwell TJ, Shah J, et al. Long-term results of a self-expanding wallstent in the treatment of urethral stricture. BJU Int 2004;94(7):1037–9.

36. Chancellor MB, Gajewski J, Ackman CF, et al. Long-term followup of the North American multicenter UroLume trial for the treatment of external detrusor-sphincter dyssynergia. J Urol 1999; 161(5):1545–50.

37. Badlani GH, Press SM, Defalco A, et al. Urolume endourethral prosthesis for the treatment of urethral stricture disease: long-term results of the North American Multicenter UroLume Trial. Urology 1995;45(5):846–56.

38. Erickson BA, McAninch JW, Eisenberg ML, et al. Management for prostate cancer treatment related posterior urethral and bladder neck stenosis with stents. J Urol 2011;185(1):198–203.

39. Besarani D, Amoroso P, Kirby R. Bladder neck contracture after radical retropubic prostatectomy. BJU Int 2004;94(9):1245–7.

40. Park R, Martin S, Goldberg JD, et al. Anastomotic strictures following radical prostatectomy: insights into incidence, effectiveness of intervention, effect on continence, and factors predisposing to occurrence. Urology 2001;57(4):742–6.

41. Anger JT, Raj GV, Delvecchio FC, et al. Anastomotic contracture and incontinence after radical prostatectomy: a graded approach to management. J Urol 2005;173(4):1143–6.

42. Yurkanin JP, Dalkin BL, Cui H. Evaluation of cold knife urethrotomy for the treatment of anastomotic stricture after radical retropubic prostatectomy. J Urol 2001;165(5):1545–8.

43. Pansadoro V, Emiliozzi P. Iatrogenic prostatic urethral strictures: classification and endoscopic treatment. Urology 1999;53(4):784–9.

44. Schlossberg S, Jordan G, Schellhammer P. Repair of obliterative vesicourethral stricture after radical prostatectomy: a technique for preservation of continence. Urology 1995;45(3):510–3.

45. Theodoros C, Katsifotis C, Stournaras P, et al. Abdomino-perineal repair of recurrent and complex bladder neck-prostatic urethra contractures. Eur Urol 2000;38(6):734–40 [discussion: 740–1].

46. Wessells H, Morey AF, McAninch JW. Obliterative vesicourethral strictures following radical

prostatectomy for prostate cancer: reconstructive armamentarium. J Urol 1998;160(4):1373–5.

47. Simonato A, Gregori A, Lissiani A, et al. Two-stage transperineal management of posterior urethral strictures or bladder neck contractures associated with urinary incontinence after prostate surgery and endoscopic treatment failures. Eur Urol 2007; 52(5):1499–504.

48. Mundy AR, Andrich DE. Posterior urethral complications of the treatment of prostate cancer. BJU Int 2012;110(3):304–25.

49. Reiss P, Pfalzgraf D, Kluth L, et al. Perineal-reanastomosis for the treatment of recurrent anastomotic strictures: outcome and patient satisfaction [abstract]. J Urol 2011;185(4):e84.

50. Kundu SD, Roehl KA, Eggener SE, et al. Potency, continence and complications in 3,477 consecutive radical retropubic prostatectomies. J Urol 2004; 172(6 Pt 1):2227–31.

51. Lepor H, Kaci L. The impact of open radical retropubic prostatectomy on continence and lower urinary tract symptoms: a prospective assessment using validated self-administered outcome instruments. J Urol 2004;171(3):1216–9.

52. Sacco E, Prayer-Galetti T, Pinto F, et al. Urinary incontinence after radical prostatectomy: incidence by definition, risk factors and temporal trend in a large series with a long-term follow-up. BJU Int 2006;97(6):1234–41.

53. Borawski K, Webster G. Long term consequences in the management of the devastated, obstructed outlet using combined Urolume stent with subsequent artificial urinary sphincter placement [abstract]. J Urol 2010;183(4):e427.

54. Sanderson KM, Penson DF, Cai J, et al. Salvage radical prostatectomy: quality of life outcome and long-term oncological control of radiorecurrent prostate cancer. J Urol 2006;176(5):2025–31 [discussion: 2031–2].

55. Stephenson AJ, Scardino PT, Bianco FJ Jr, et al. Morbidity and functional outcomes of salvage radical prostatectomy for locally recurrent prostate cancer after radiation therapy. J Urol 2004; 172(6 Pt 1):2239–43.

56. Eltahawy E, Gur U, Virasoro R, et al. Management of recurrent anastomotic stenosis following radical prostatectomy using holmium laser and steroid injection. BJU Int 2008;102(7):796–8.

57. Vanni AJ, Zinman LN, Buckley JC. Radial urethrotomy and intralesional mitomycin C for the management of recurrent bladder neck contractures. J Urol 2011;186(1):156–60.

58. Hou JC, Landas S, Wang CY, et al. Instillation of mitomycin C after transurethral resection of bladder cancer impairs wound healing: an animal model. Anticancer Res 2011;31(3):929–32.

59. Doherty AP, Trendell-Smith N, Stirling R, et al. Perivesical fat necrosis after adjuvant intravesical chemotherapy. BJU Int 1999;83(4):420–3.

60. Oddens JR, van der Meijden AP, Sylvester R. One immediate postoperative instillation of chemotherapy in low risk Ta, T1 bladder cancer patients. Is it always safe? Eur Urol 2004;46(3): 336–8.

61. Moran DE, Moynagh MR, Alzanki M, et al. Anaphylaxis at image-guided epidural pain block secondary to corticosteroid compound. Skeletal Radiol 2012;41(10):1317–8.

Tips for Successful Open Surgical Reconstruction of Posterior Urethral Disruption Injuries

Joel Gelman, MD

KEYWORDS

- Posterior urethral disruption • Posterior urethroplasty • Pelvic fracture urethral distraction defect
- Urethral stricture • Urethral reconstruction

KEY POINTS

- After suprapubic tube placement, delayed open urethral reconstruction with excision and primary anastomosis via a perineal approach is the standard of care for the initial treatment of pelvic fracture urethral disruption injuries and treatment after failed endoscopic realignment.
- Before urethroplasty, accurate assessment of the defect is reliably obtained with a retrograde urethrogram and simultaneous antegrade cystourethrogram with contrast instillation through the tip of the scope positioned in the prostatic urethra.
- Vascular testing before urethral reconstruction may identify patients who are at risk for ischemic anterior urethral stenosis and who may benefit from penile revascularization before posterior urethroplasty.
- When performed using the proper technique, posterior urethroplasty offers a high success rate and a low complication rate.

INTRODUCTION: NATURE OF THE PROBLEM

Pelvic fracture trauma in males, often secondary to motor vehicle trauma or pelvic crush injuries, can be associated with injuries to the posterior urethra, especially where there is pubic symphysis diastasis or there are displaced inferomedial pubic bone fractures.[1] When the pelvis is fractured, the patient is often found to have blood at the urethral meatus. Additional symptoms and signs of urethral injury include bladder distension, inability to void, perineal hematoma, and possibly a high riding prostate on digital rectal examination.

A retrograde urethrogram (RUG) is indicated when a urethral injury is suspected and typically shows extravasation as a result of a partial tear, or more often, a complete disruption. The term prostatomembranous disruption is often used to describe these injuries, and this terminology suggests that the transection occurs at the junction of the prostatic and membranous portions of the posterior urethra. However, more recent studies, including an autopsy review of male patients who sustained pelvic fracture–related urethral injuries and died of associated multiple trauma, revealed that the injuries are generally bulbomembranous and distal to the urogenital diaphragm.[2] There can be proximal or distal extension, but the injury generally remains distal to the verumontanum of the prostate. Continence after repair is maintained

Funding Sources: None.
Conflicts of Interest: None.
Department of Urology, Center for Reconstructive Urology, University of California, Irvine Medical Center, Orange, CA 92868, USA
E-mail address: jgelman@uci.edu

Urol Clin N Am 40 (2013) 381–392
http://dx.doi.org/10.1016/j.ucl.2013.04.007

primarily by the proximal bladder neck. However, in many patients, there is also a significant rhabdosphincter contribution, as shown by video urodynamic testing after reconstruction.[3]

The standard management approach is suprapubic tube placement and delayed posterior urethral reconstruction. Alternatively, primary realignment can be performed, which is discussed by Wessels and colleagues, elsewhere in this issue. Should this option fail, the definitive treatment is then delayed posterior urethroplasty with excision and primary anastomosis via a perineal approach.

SURGICAL TECHNIQUE: PREOPERATIVE PLANNING
3-Month Delay

We wait 3 months from the time of injury or catheter removal in cases of failed primary realignment before performing urethroplasty, to allow time for the initial extravasation to heal, hematoma to resolve, and the extent of the injury to become clearly defined. It has been shown that after manipulation, several months of urethral rest is required for before anterior urethral strictures become clearly defined.[4] When there is a pelvic fracture–associated injury to the posterior urethra, initial imaging reveals extravasation, whereas imaging 3 months after injury typically confirms no extravasation and clear delineation of the location and length of the defect. Recent publications indicate that the delay is often a minimum of 3 to 6 months. However, the interval between initial injury and urethroplasty can exceed 1 year when there are associated injuries.[5–9] A recently presented abstract indicated that urethral reconstruction less than 6 weeks after the injury may be associated with results similar to when there is a delay of 3 or more months.[10] However, there are no recent publications suggesting that a delay of less than 3 months is appropriate, and the current delay of no less than 3 months is the current published minimum period of urethral rest.

Suprapubic Urinary Diversion

Suprapubic tube urinary diversion always precedes urethroplasty. The ideal suprapubic tube is no less than 16 French, midline, and 2 fingerbreadths above the pubic symphysis. However, patients are often initially managed with tubes that are far lateral to the midline or just above the symphysis. In some cases, very small caliber pigtail catheters are placed (**Fig. 1**). When patients are referred for posterior urethral reconstruction, and have tubes of inadequate caliber or if the tube is not in the ideal position, it is our preference to percutaneously place a new 16-Fr tube. This

procedure is generally performed as soon as possible when the caliber is small, and no less than 1 month before urethroplasty so there will be an established stable tract at the time of surgery. Small caliber pigtail catheters are especially prone to encrustation and urinary retention. Moreover, catheters placed just above the symphysis are more uncomfortable than catheters placed in a higher position away from the bone. The main benefit of having the suprapubic tube midline well above the symphysis with an established tract is that this facilitates the surgery and prevents the need for a temporary vesicostomy. During posterior urethroplasty with the patient in the lithotomy position, after perineal exposure is achieved and the urethra is transected, a metal sound is generally advanced through the established tract, and perineal dissection proceeds toward the tip of the sound until the sound can be seen and advanced into the perineum. When the caliber of the tract is inadequate, sounds do not advance without dilation at the time of the surgery. This situation can be associated with bleeding and compromise of the tract. When the tube is just above the bone, a very acute angle is needed to advance the sound through the bladder neck. Moreover, when the tract is lateral to the midline, the rigid sound cannot be reliably advanced medially toward the midline bladder neck and then distally along the posterior urethra. One option is to create a temporary vesicostomy. However, this procedure adds considerable time and morbidity to the reconstructive surgery and therefore this is not our preference.

PREOPERATIVE URETHRAL EVALUATION: CYSTOSCOPY

Before definitive urethral reconstruction, urethroscopy, antegrade cystoscopy, and a simultaneous antegrade cystourethrogram and RUG together provide a definitive diagnosis of the length and location of the defect. One common imaging technique is for the bladder to be filled with contrast by gravity through the suprapubic tube and for a RUG to be performed as the patient is asked to perform the Valsalva maneuver and attempt to void. As the patient attempts to void, if the bladder neck opens, there is filling of the posterior urethra proximal to the obliteration, and the length of the defect is determined (**Fig. 2**A). However, in many cases, the patient cannot relax to void when the urethra is obliterated and contrast is being injected through the penis. When the bladder neck is intact, the appearance is as shown in **Fig. 2**B. The distance between the bladder and the distal end of the defect is not the length of

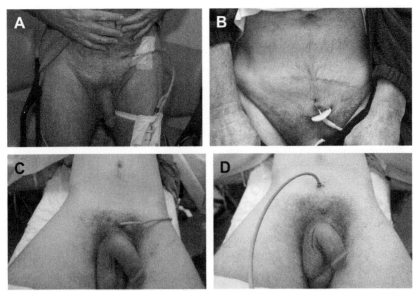

Fig. 1. (A) Laterally placed suprapubic tube. (B) Small pigtail catheter of inadequate caliber. (C) Suprapubic tube placed below the ideal location. (D) Suprapubic tube repositioned midline 2 finger breaths above the midline pubic symphysis.

the distraction defect, because the prostatic urethra is not visualized. In a recent study in which the goal was to determine if the type of urethroplasty could be predicted based on certain features from the preoperative imaging, 38% of the 100 study patients evaluated with a Valsalva cystourethrogram and RUG were excluded because there was no visualization of the urethra below the bladder neck.[4]

Our preferred approach is to first perform antegrade cystoscopy with the patient prepared and draped in the oblique position after a 35 × 43 cm (14 × 17 inch) scout film is obtained to confirm proper position and penetration. Some patients develop bladder calculi, and when identified, the stones can be removed before urethroplasty. The bladder neck is then inspected for coaptation. An open bladder neck at rest suggests that there may be an increased incidence of incontinence

after urethral reconstruction. Iselin and Webster identified 15 patients who sustained pelvic fracture urethral injuries and had an open bladder neck at rest.[11] Six were continent and 8 were incontinent after urethroplasty. However, MacDiarmid and colleagues[12] identified 4 patients who had an open bladder neck at rest, and all of these patients were continent after surgery. Although some surgeons occasionally perform bladder neck reconstruction at the time of posterior urethroplasty,[13] most reconstructive urologists do not perform simultaneous bladder neck surgery, given the observation that an open bladder neck at rest does not reliably predict postoperative incontinence. When we observe an open bladder neck at rest, the patient is counseled that there may be an increased incidence of postoperative incontinence, but this finding does not influence our management.

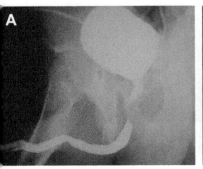
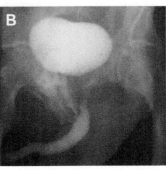

Fig. 2. (A) After the bladder is filled with contrast through the suprapubic tube, an RUG is performed as the patient is asked to attempt to void. If the bladder neck opens, contrast fills the prostatic urethra, and the membranous urethral defect is seen. (B) When the bladder neck does not open, the length of the defect cannot be determined accurately.

PREOPERATIVE URETHRAL EVALUATION: URETHRAL IMAGING

Once the scope is advanced through the bladder neck, the location of the proximal aspect of the injury is noted, and this is almost always distal to the verumontanum of the prostate within the membranous urethra. With the tip of the scope at the level of the obliteration, full-strength contrast is injected, which then back fills the posterior urethra and bladder. Simultaneously, an RUG is performed. Our preferred technique for performing an RUG is to place a gauze around the coronal sulcus to place the penis on stretch, and inject contract through a cone-shaped Taylor adaptor (Cook Urological Incorporated, Spencer, IN, USA) connected to a 60-mL syringe filled with full-strength contrast (**Fig. 3**). Many published textbooks advocate the advancement of a catheter into the fossa navicularis and inflation of the balloon with 1 to 3 mL of contrast for form a seal. However, the balloon caliber of catheters of several different sizes when inflated with only 2 mL of fluid or air is approximately 59 French, and the normal caliber of the adult anterior urethra is approximately 30 French, except at the level of the urethral meatus and fossa navicularis, where the caliber is approximately 24 French (**Fig. 4**A). Therefore, the balloon dilates the normal distal anterior urethra, which can be associated with considerable pain and even stricture disease of the fossa navicularis. We have seen patients referred for strictures initially limited to the bulbar urethra who then developed narrow caliber fossa strictures after undergoing painful urethral imaging when the technique included balloon inflation within the fossa navicularis (see **Fig. 4**B).

Simultaneous antegrade and retrograde imaging and endoscopy performed with proper technique clearly defines the length and location of the defect. Other imaging modalities that can be used include magnetic resonance imaging and ultrasonography.[14] However, we have never found an indication to perform these additional tests. Fluoroscopy offers the advantage of dynamic real-time imaging. However, disadvantages include a reduced field of view and decreased resolution compared with conventional radiographs. We prefer flat plate imaging using digital cassettes that can be digitized and stored electronically and also printed on 14 × 17 film. Although magnification and positioning can influence the scale, we have observed that the length of the obliteration measured directly on the film accurately corresponds to the length of the defect at the time of surgery. Most defects are 1 to 3 cm in length and within the membranous urethra, with possible extension into the most proximal bulbar urethra. Although pelvic fracture trauma typically injures the posterior urethra, if there is also straddle trauma at the time of the pelvic fracture, the injury can be to the bulbar urethra. The specific location of the injury can influence the management. For example, a man who sustained pelvic fracture trauma during a race car accident was found to have significant extravasation on an RUG on the day of the injury and was managed with a laterally placed suprapubic tube. Delayed imaging and antegrade cystoscopy confirmed a proximal bulbar urethral defect and a normal membranous urethra (**Fig. 5**). Although both traumatic proximal bulbar and membranous disruptions are managed with excision and primary anastomosis, bulbar urethroplasty does not require antegrade access to facilitate identification of the patent proximal segment. If the injury were membranous, then a new midline suprapubic tube would have been placed to facilitate subsequent antegrade access to the proximal segment at the time of posterior urethroplasty. However, because antegrade access is not required for bulbar urethroplasty, the placement of a new midline tube was not required.

PREOPERATIVE VASCULAR EVALUATION

The anterior urethra has a dual blood supply, with an additional minor contribution provided by

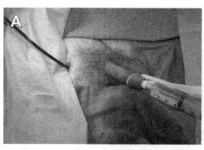
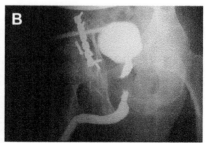

Fig. 3. (*A*) A RUG is performed as contrast is simultaneously injected into the posterior urethra through the flexible cystoscope, with the tip in the distal prostatic urethra. (*B*) Imaging accurately shows the length and location of the defect.

A

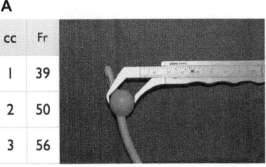

cc	Fr
1	39
2	50
3	56

B

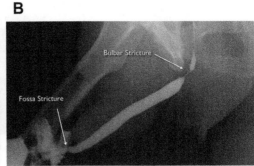

Fig. 4. (*A*) Catheter balloon inflation with only 1 to 3 cm³ of air or fluid is associated with balloon inflation well beyond the normal caliber of the normal fossa navicularis. (*B*) Repeat RUG showing in addition to the previously seen bulbar stricture, a new fossa navicularis stricture, which developed after an RUG was performed using fossa balloon inflation technique.

perforating vessels between the corpora cavernosa and the corpus spongiosum. The bulbar arteries enter the corpus spongiosum at the level of the most proximal bulbar urethra and provide antegrade flow to the corpus spongiosum of the anterior urethra. In addition, the dorsal arteries course within the neurovascular strictures along the dorsal aspect of the penis superficial to the corporal bodies and supply the glans penis, which is the distal expansion of the corpus spongiosum. This anatomy provides a secondary blood supply to the anterior urethra as the blood courses in retrograde fashion along the corpus spongiosum. When the urethra is completely transected at the departure of the anterior urethra, any patent bulbar arteries are ligated or cauterized. The anterior urethra then survives as a flap based on the retrograde dorsal artery contribution in addition to perforating vessels. Although results are unpublished, it has been observed by several reconstructive urologists that in rare cases, long-segment bulbar strictures developed as

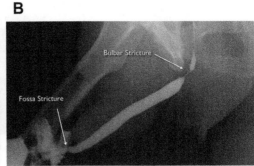

Fig. 5. Simultaneous antegrade and retrograde urethral imaging showing a bulbar urethral obliteration, further confirmed with antegrade cystoscopy.

an ischemic complication of posterior urethroplasty. The mechanism of the ischemic stenosis was presumed to be compromise of the bulbar artery supply during surgery in patients who suffered perineal trauma that compromised dorsal artery supply. We have observed cases of ischemic stenosis in patients with hypospadias who developed discreet bulbar strictures and were treated with a urethral stent.[15] Before stent placement, these patients were noted on urethroscopy to have a normal caliber anterior urethra distal to the bulbar stricture. After stent placement, they developed severe panurethral disease. This finding makes sense anatomically because hypospadias and corrective surgery are associated with a compromise of the corpus spongiosum distally and the associated retrograde blood supply to the more proximal anterior urethra. These patients were likely bulbar dependent, and stent expansion compromised the antegrade bulbar artery flow distal to the stent. Therefore, in addition to antegrade cystoscopy and contrast imaging, we perform a preoperative vascular evaluation to identify patients who have severe arterial inflow compromise to both dorsal arteries, and perform penile revascularization before urethral reconstruction in selected cases. Penile revascularization provides a microvascular anastomosis of the inferior epigastric artery to the dorsal artery of the penis (**Fig. 6**).

Erectile dysfunction and pudendal vascular injuries are highly associated with pelvic fracture urethral disruptions. In a study by Shenfeld and colleagues,[16] 25 patients who sustained traumatic posterior urethral disruptions were evaluated with nocturnal penile tumescence testing. Eighteen patients (72%) were found to have erectile dysfunction, and these patients underwent a penile duplex with pharmacologic erection that revealed arterial inflow impairment in 5 of 18

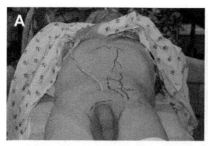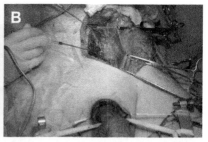

Fig. 6. Inferior epigastric artery to dorsal artery penile revascularization, shown after skin marking (A) and durin surgery (B).

patients. The remaining patients were considered to have a neurogenic cause of their erectile dysfunction. Davies and colleagues[17] performed a penile duplex testing on 56 men who sustained posterior urethral disruptions, and identified 25 men with vascular compromise. These patients underwent arteriogram. Twenty-one had reconstitution of 1 or both pudendals, and 4 did not. These 4 patients underwent revascularization before urethral reconstruction, and no patient developed ischemic stenosis after surgery. A limitation of this study is that it is not known if any of these patients would have developed stenosis if reconstruction had been performed without prior revascularization. This is an area of controversy. However, we believe that vascular testing and revascularization in selected cases may be justified based on the anatomic principals and the available data. Moreover, revascularization often successfully treats the erectile dysfunction associated with pelvic fracture injuries.[18]

POSTERIOR URETHRAL RECONSTRUCTION: PREPARATION AND PATIENT POSITIONING

Before surgery, which we generally perform approximately 3 months after injury, patients are placed in high lithotomy during a physical examination to assess hip flexion and ability to tolerate this position. Some patients may have unresolved back or other orthopedic problems, which may then be exacerbated by prolonged lithotomy positioning. In our series of 85 patients, the longest delay was 19 months. This patient had severe compromise of hip flexion, which persisted more than 12 months after the injury. With ongoing physical therapy, mobility returned to normal, and positioning was safely accomplished without compromise. A urine culture is sent the week before surgery. The specimen is obtained by clamping the suprapubic tube, and then unclamping the tube 20 minutes later over a specimen container. The sample is then obtained directly from the suprapubic tube and not the drainage

bag. Any mixed growth is separately culture Patients are admitted the day before surgery fc dual coverage antibiotics. Our protocol is t administer piperacillin/tazobactam and tobram cin, but adjust the antibiotics if indicated base on the culture result. No patient has suffered th complication of a perineal infection, which ca be associated with urethral compromise and stri ture development.

Although some reconstructive urologists prefe a low lithotomy position, in many centers and i our institution, exaggerated lithotomy positionin is preferred. This position can be associate with severe complications, including neur praxia, compartment syndrome, and rhabdomyc losis.[19–21] Neuropraxia is usually not permanen Sensory deficits are more common than mote impairment, and the risk of a positioning complica tion is related to the time in lithotomy. One form c exaggerated lithotomy, often used for perine prostatectomy, places hips under considerab flexion so that the thighs are parallel to the bac and the floor. In a study by Holzbeierlein an colleagues,[22] of 111 men who underwent a radic perineal prostatectomy in this extreme lithotom position with a mean duration of less than 3 hour 23 (21%) suffered a positioning complication. C these 23 patients, 17 had symptoms at the tim of discharge, and 6 required physical therap support for ambulation.

We use a Skytron Custom 6000 table modifie by Jordan to offer an electronic pelvic tilt mecha nism to cradle the pelvis as an alternative t raising the buttocks and placing a beanbag sup port (**Fig. 7**A). In addition, stirrups are modifie to provide additional extension so that hip an knee flexion is reduced. Foam padding is place along the dorsal feet and anterior legs to even distribute the pressure (see **Fig. 7**B). We previ ously used gel pads, and found a significant reduced incidence of temporary (24-hour t 48-hour) dorsal foot numbness after a change c the use of the softer foam. Extreme flexion c the hips and knees is avoided, and the boot

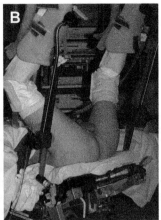
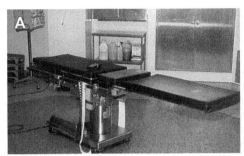

Fig. 7. (*A*) Modified Skytron Custom 6000 surgical table with pelvic tilt mechanism (highlighted in *yellow*), (*B*) patient placed in exaggerated lithotomy position.

re tilted so that there is no pressure on the alves.

POSTERIOR URETHRAL RECONSTRUCTION: SURGICAL TECHNIQUE

Exposure

A midline perineal incision is 1 option. We prefer an inverted Y-shaped λ incision to obtain generous exposure (**Fig. 8**A). This incision is carried medial to the ischial tuberosities posteriorly and along the median scrotal raphe. Dissection then proceeds sharply though the subcutaneous fat longitudinally along the midline until the bulbopongiosus muscle is encountered. The Jordan-Simpson perineal retractor is used to facilitate exposure as shown in **Fig. 8**B. Although other retractors are commercially available such as the Lone Star retractor, advantages of the Jordan retractor include fixation of the ring and the ability to use a variety of different specialized blades in

addition to the hooks used in the Lone Star system. In addition, tilt ratchets facilitate lateral retraction to facilitate exposure. The bulbospongiosus muscle is then divided and retracted laterally to expose the bulb. The bulb is detached from the perineal body, and we find that the use of a bipolar cautery facilitates this dissection and maintains hemostasis to the extent that suction is seldom required. The urethra is then circumferentially mobilized from the penoscrotal junction distally to the departure of the anterior urethra proximally (see **Fig. 8**C). This is performed sharply without the use of right angle clamps, which can tear the corpus spongiosum. The bulbar arteries are transected and cauterized if patent.

Several recent articles have described bulbar artery–sparing anastomotic anterior urethroplasty.[23,24] Although the use of artery-sparing surgery during posterior urethral reconstruction has not been published, a recent abstract[25] described the successful use of this

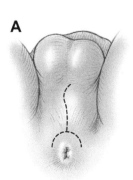
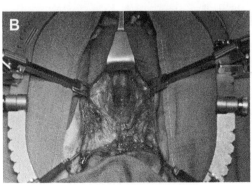
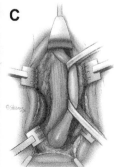

Fig. 8. (*A*) λ Incision with the patient in the exaggerated lithotomy position. (*B*) Jordan-Simpson perineal retractor is used to facilitate exposure of the corpus spongiosum. (*C*) The corpus spongiosum is circumferentially mobilized along the bulbar urethra.

technique in 9 patients. Intraoperative ultrasonography was performed, and the artery with the strongest signal was preserved. No patient developed a recurrent stricture with a mean follow-up of 10 months. This finding may possibly represent a future modification of operative technique.

Proximal Exposure and Scar Excision

After transection of the urethra, unless preoperative imaging suggests very short segment obliteration, we routinely separate the corporal bodies at the level of the triangular ligament and retract them laterally to improve proximal exposure and facilitate excision of the scar tissue, which is generally whitish and firm.

The suprapubic tube is then removed and a curved metal sound is advanced through the established tract into the bladder and then through the bladder neck, guided by feel, until the impulse of the tip of the sound can be palpated in the perineum as the sound is manipulated. This tech nique guides the dissection in the appropriat direction toward the patent proximal urethra. On option is to advance a Van Buren sound. Althoug these instruments are often readily available an familiar to most urologists, the fact that the instru ment is curved only at the tip and tapered to more pointed tip relative to the shaft of the instru ment renders these instruments poorly suited t use in posterior urethroplasty, especially when a exaggerated lithotomy position is used. Howeve the semicircular Haygrove sound is designed t best follow the path from the suprapubic acces to the membranous urethra (**Fig. 9**A, B). Th caliber is not greater than 16 to 18 Fr, and there fore, no tract dilation is required if the indwellin suprapubic tube was 16 Fr. In addition, the tip i curved and smooth. However, in some cases the tip of the sound may not be palpable. This sit uation may be because of the presence of ver dense scar or malposition of the sound. If dissec tion proceeds in the wrong direction, what i

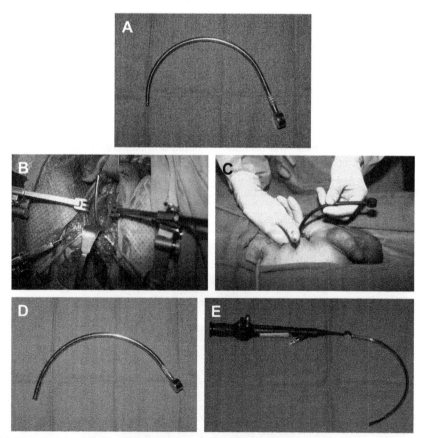

Fig. 9. (A) Solid Haygrove sound. (B) After dissection of the obliterative scar, the tip of the sound (placed through the suprapubic tract) can then be advanced through the patent proximal urethra into the perineum. (C) Temporary vesicostomy in a patient with a laterally placed suprapubic tube. (D) Gelman visualizing posterior urethra sound. (E) Flexible scope advanced through the hollow visualizing sound.

ntered may be the bladder or the posterior ure-
ıra proximal to the distal aspect of the patent ure-
ıra. This situation may lead to postoperative
ıcontinence or restenosis. The limitation of a solid
ɔund is that it is guided blindly. If a flexible cysto-
cope is used, the scope can be guided under
ʲrect vision. However, because the active scope
eflection is limited only to the tip of the scope, it
ıay be difficult to advance the tip of the scope
ɔ the proper position, especially when the patient
. in high lithotomy and the surgeon is positioned
t the level of the perineum. To prevent the possi-
ility of false passages, some surgeons perform
gid antegrade cystoscopy before the patient is
repared and draped in the exaggerated lithotomy
ɔsition, advance the scope through the bladder
eck and prostatic urethra, then palpate the peri-
eum to determine if the tip of the scope is
alpable or not.[26] When the tip of the scope is
ɔt palpable, or if the suprapubic tube is laterally
ɔcated, a temporary vesicostomy is created
efore lithotomy positioning and then taken
own after the completion of the repair (see
ig. 9C). It was determined that the creation of
ıe vesicostomy allows the surgeon to palpably
ʲentify the bladder neck before instrumentation
f the posterior urethra, and that this maneuver
liminates the occurrence of false passages and
ıe misanastomosis of the anterior urethra to sites
ther than the apical prostatic urethra. This ma-
euver adds considerable time and morbidity to
ıe surgery.

For this reason, we prefer to always proceed
ʲith a midline suprapubic tube, even if this
equires placement of a new tube no less than
   month before urethroplasty to allow time for
ıe tract to mature, and use a new visualizing
ɔund (Gelman Urethral Sound, CS Surgical) (see
ɨig. 9D). This sound has a contour similar to the
ʲaygrove sound, but is hollow, allowing a flexible
ʲystoscope to be advanced through the sound
ʲee Fig. 9E). The tip of the sound or the tip of
ʲe cystoscope can then be directed to the obliter-
ıtion under direct vision. An additional advantage
ʲ that the light from the scope can be seen to
ʲrther guide the dissection. Before the develop-
ʲent of the visualizing sound, 2 of 9 patients
equired a temporary vesicostomy at the time of
econstruction. Subsequently, 76 patients (ages
ʲ–77 years) underwent reconstruction, (including
ʲ pediatric patients, and 14 patients who had
ʲnsuccessful procedures before referral), and
ʲ of 76 patients required a temporary vesicostomy.
ʲn every case, the sound could be directed to the
ʲroper position under direct vision. It is our expe-
ʲence that the visualizing posterior urethral sound
ʲreatly facilitates the reliable identification and

dissection of the proximal segment during posterior urethral reconstruction. With the use of this
device, the open dissection can be limited to the
perineal exploration, even in pediatric and difficult
cases. One disadvantage of the sound is that the
outside diameter is greater than the outside diameter of the solid Haygrove sound, and the solid
sound can be manipulated more easily. Therefore,
we continue to use the solid sound when the tip
can be readily palpated in the perineum. Although
the larger-diameter hollow sound does not
advance as easily though the suprapubic tract
when 16-Fr to 18-Fr indwelling tubes are used
before surgery, the tip of the flexible cystoscope
can be first advanced into the bladder, and the
sound can then be advanced over the scope using
the scope as the equivalent of a guide wire.

The most complex portion of posterior urethral
reconstruction is the proximal exposure and
dissection after transection of the urethra. One option is to sharply incise scar tissue, advance a nasal
speculum through the scar, and place J-shaped
sutures through the speculum to initiate the anastomosis.[27] It is our preference to excise the scar
tissue until normal healthy tissue is encountered.
Supple tissue more readily everts, bringing the
mucosa forward from deep within the pelvis during
the placement of the first several sutures, and this
facilitates the placement of subsequent sutures.
Our objective is to achieve the proximal preplace-
ment of 10 to 12 3-0 absorbable monofilament
sutures. We alternate using violet PDS and clear
Monocryl to help maintain orientation at the time
of the completion of the anastomosis.

Infrapubectomy

In cases in which the scar is especially dense and
the defect is long, it is possible that the tip of the
sound is not palpable, and the light of the cystoscope is not seen even if it is confirmed using
the visualizing sound that the tip of the sound
and scope are in the appropriate position at the
distal aspect of the patent posterior urethra. In
these cases, scar tissue just below the midline
symphysis is excised sharply in a 1-cm-diameter
to 2-cm-diameter area. As the scar is excised,
the dissection extends deep into the pelvis, and
it is in these cases in particular that infrapubectomy is often required. After the separation of the
corporal bodies at the level of the triangular ligament and lateral retraction, the dorsal vein is
then mobilized and ligated, exposing the midline
symphysis pubis. Periosteal elevators are then
used to sweep the medial crura laterally and
free the undersurface of the bone from adherent
tissue. Kerrison rongeurs provide controlled bone

removal, which widens the exposure and facilitates further proximal dissection. Moreover, the separation of the corpora and infrapubectomy provide a more direct route for the urethra to course, and this facilitates a tension-free repair.

Additional Maneuvers

Some investigators have reported that in addition to distal mobilization, crural separation, and infrapubectomy, supracrural corporal rerouting was required to achieve an acceptable amount of tension in select cases.[28] This technique seems to be associated with a high rate of restenosis. In a recently published combined series of 142 cases, 4 underwent rerouting and 3 of these patients (75%) developed restenosis.[9] Other surgeons never find supracrural rerouting to be a beneficial maneuver. It is often stated that the objective is a tension-free anastomosis. This procedure is not necessary because there is normally a certain amount of innate tension along the corpus spongiosum. For this reason, when the urethra is transected, there is generally some retraction of the distal segment. Our goal is not a tension-free anastomosis, but rather an anastomosis without unacceptable tension that would lead to tethering of the penis during erections or separation of the anastomosis. We have never encountered a case in which supracrural rerouting was required.

Another option in complex cases in which there is a large gap is a transpubic approach.[29–31] We have never found this technique necessary, and more recent reports[32] confirm that infrapubectomy generally provides adequate proximal exposure in complex cases. Moreover, tissue transfer with flaps or grafts has been reported as an option to bridge longer defects.[28] This procedure seems to have been performed mostly in older series, and recent reports do not support the use of or need for tissue transfer. It is fortunate that excision and primary anastomosis can reliably be achieved during posterior urethral reconstruction, given that tube flaps and grafts are generally associated with a high failure rate, and the tissues surrounding the membranous urethra deep within the pelvis proximal to the triangular ligament do not represent a suitable bed for graft spread fixation.

Anastomosis

Once the proximal sutures are placed along a widely patent proximal segment surrounded by pink healthy mucosa proximally, and flexible cystoscopy further confirms that the opening is distal to the verumontanum at the appropriate location, the distal segment is dorsally spatulated and calibrated using bougies à boule. The caliber

should be greater than 30 Fr. The anastomosis then completed as a stenting catheter is placed It is our preference to use a 14-Fr soft silicon catheter. A small TLS train is placed deep adjace to the corpus spongiosum deep to the bulbospon giosus muscle, which is then reapproximate along the ventral midline, and a second fl 7-mm drain is placed superficial to the muscl The incision is then closed in 2 layers with absorb able suture and a clear dressing is placed. N compressive dressing is required.

Postoperative Care

Our protocol is to maintain the stenting urethr catheter and the suprapubic tube urinary diversic for 3 weeks, and then perform a voiding cystou ethrogram by removing the stenting cathete filling the bladder with contract by gravity installa tion, and then obtaining a film during urination. I the rare case of extravasation, a new stentin catheter is replaced and a repeat study is pe formed the next week. Other surgeons favor cath eter removal without postoperative imaging.[33] I most cases, the force of stream is excellent, ar the suprapubic tube is then removed. If the strea is not weak, the tube is plugged and the patient instructed to unplug the tube at home if unable t urinate and to check residuals by unplugging th tube after micturition. One possible reason fc voiding difficulty is neurogenic bladder dysfunc tion related to the initial injury, especially if ther is associated back trauma. Several months afte tube removal, flexible urethroscopy is performe to definitively confirm wide patency of the repai Patients are then encouraged to have a baselin flow rate and postvoid residual assessment, an then to have this repeated annually. There is lack of consensus regarding appropriate follow up after surgery.

Outcomes

In our series of 85 patients, before referral, 1 underwent failed endoscopic treatment and 1 underwent failed open surgery. At the time of su gery, 19 patients underwent infrapubectomy, an no patient required supracrural rerouting. N patient required transfusion, and the only persis tent neuropraxia was in 1 patient, who had persis tent tingling of the toes, which resolved afte several months. At the time of urethroscop 4 months after surgery, 2 patients were noted t have medium caliber narrowing. One of thes patients underwent dilation 2 years after surger and the other was observed and never require treatment. This finding corresponds to a succes rate of 97.6% success, defined as durable wid atency of the repair and with no further treatment equired.

Other series report a similar success rate for dults, adolescents, and children, and this indi-ates that a stricture recurrence after a properly erformed posterior urethroplasty should be a are event.[32,34] Of the patients who presented to ur center after failed surgery, the recurrence was ften within days or weeks, suggesting that these rere technical failures, likely because of inade-uate scar excision with an anastomosis to a widely atent segment of proximal urethral mucosa. urther suggesting that technical inexperience of ne surgeon is likely the most common cause of ailure is the fact that these patients usually have successful outcome with the same technique of xcisional repair when the revision surgery is per-ormed by a specialist in urethral reconstruction. Published studies from referral centers confirm nat when open repair fails, excision and primary nastomosis still remains the procedure of choice nd when properly performed, offers a high suc-ess rate.[35,36] Delayed posterior urethral disruption njuries are highly amenable to successful recon-truction with excisional posterior urethroplasty ia a perineal approach.

REFERENCES

1. Basta C, Blackmore CC, Wessells H. Predicting urethral injury from pelvic fracture trauma patterns in male patients with blunt trauma. J Urol 2007; 177:571–5.

2. Mouraviev VB, Santucci RA. Cadaveric anatomy of pelvic fracture urethral distraction injury: most injuries are distal to the external urinary sphincter. J Urol 2005;173(3):869–72.

3. Whitson JM, McAninch JW, Tanagho EA, et al. Mechanism of continence after repair of posterior urethral disruption: evidence of rhabdosphincter activity. J Urol 2008;179:1035–9.

4. Terlecki RP, Steele MC, Valadez CM, et al. Urethral rest: role and rationale in preparation for anterior urethroplasty. Urology 2011;77(6):1477–81.

5. Andrich DE, O'Malley KJ, Summerton DJ, et al. The type of urethroplasty for a pelvic fracture urethral distraction defect cannot be predicted preopera-tively. J Urol 2003;170:464–7.

6. Tunc HM, Tefekli AH, Kaplancan T, et al. Delayed repair of post-traumatic posterior urethral distraction injuries: long-term results. Urology 2000;55(6): 837–41.

7. Koraitim MM. On the art of anastomotic posterior urethroplasty: a 27-year experience. J Urol 2005; 173:135–9.

8. Fu Q, Zhand J, Sa YL, et al. Transperineal bulbopro-static anastomosis in patients with simple traumatic posterior urethral strictures: a retrospective study from a referral urethral center. Urology 2009;74(5): 1132–7.

9. Kizer WS, Armenakas NA, Brandes SB, et al. Simpli-fied reconstruction of posterior urethral disruption defects: limited role of supracrural rerouting. J Urol 2007;177:1378–82.

10. Gomez RG, Bonomo J, Marchetti P, et al. Timing for reconstruction of pelvic fracture urethral disruption injuries: do we have to wait three months? J Urol 2011;184(4) [abstract 103].

11. Iselin CE, Webster GD. The significance of the open bladder neck associated with pelvic fracture urethral distraction defects. J Urol 1999;162:347–51.

12. MacDiarmid S, Rosario D, Chapple CR. The impor-tance of accurate assessment and conservative management of the open bladder neck in patients with post-pelvic fracture membranous urethral distraction defects. Br J Urol 1995;75:65–7.

13. Khoriatim MM. Assessment and management of an open bladder neck at posterior urethroplasty. Urology 2010;76(2):476–9.

14. Oh MM, Jin MH, Sung DJ, et al. Magnetic resonance urethrography to assess obliterative posterior ure-thral stricture: comparison to retrograde urethrogra-phy with voiding cystourethrography. J Urol 2010; 183:603–7.

15. Rodriguez E, Gelman J. Pan-urethral strictures can develop as a complication of UroLume placement for bulbar stricture disease in patients with hypospa-dias. Urology 2006;67(6):1290.

16. Shenfeld OZ, Kiselforf D, Gofrit ON, et al. The inci-dence and causes of erectile dysfunction after pelvic fractures associated with posterior urethral disruption. J Urol 2003;169:2173–6.

17. Davies TO, Colen LB, Cowan N, et al. Preoperative vascular evaluation of patients with pelvic fracture urethral distraction defects (PFUDD). J Urol 2009; 181(4):29.

18. Zuckerman JM, McCammon KA, Tisdale BE, et al. Outcome of penile revascularization for arteriogenic erectile dysfunction after pelvic fracture urethral injuries. Urology 2012;80(6):1369–74.

19. Angermeier KW, Jordan GH. Complications of the exaggerated lithotomy position: a review of 177 cases. J Urol 1994;151:866–8.

20. Bildsten SA, Dmochowski RR, Spindel MR, et al. The risk of rhabdomyolysis and acute renal failure with the patient in the exaggerated lithotomy position. J Urol 1994;152:1970–2.

21. Anema JG, Morey AF, McAninch JW, et al. Compli-cations related to the high lithotomy position during urethral reconstruction. J Urol 2000;164:360–3.

22. Holzbeierlein JM, Langenstroer P, Porter HJ, et al. Case selection and outcome of radical perineal prostatectomy in localized prostate cancer. Int Braz J Urol 2003;29(4):291–9.

23. Jordan JH, Eltahawy EA, Virasoro R. The technique of vessel sparing excision and primary anastomosis for proximal bulbous urethral reconstruction. J Urol 2007;177:1799–802.

24. Andrich DE, Mundy AR. Non-transecting anastomotic bulbar urethroplasty: a preliminary report. BJU Int 2011;109:1090–4.

25. Gomez RG, Marchetti P, Catalan G. Bulbar artery sparing during reconstruction of pelvic fracture urethral distraction defects. J Urol 2010;183(4) [abstract 1226].

26. Jordan GH, McCammon K. Surgery of the penis and urethra. In: Wein AJ, Kavoussi LR, Novick AC, et al, editors. Campbell-Walsh urology. 10th edition. Philadelphia: WB Saunders; 2012. p. 956–1000.

27. Carr LK, Webster GD. Posterior urethral reconstruction. Atlas Urol Clin N Am 1997;5(1):125–37.

28. Webster GD, Sihelnik S. The management of strictures of the membranous urethra. J Urol 1985;134: 469–73.

29. Waterhouse K, Abrahams JI, Gruber H, et al. The transpubic approach to the lower urinary tract. J Urol 1973;109(3):486–90.

30. Koraitim MM. The lessons of 145 posttraumatic posterior urethral strictures treated in 17 years. J Urol 1995;153(1):63–6.

31. Pratap A, Agrawal CS, Tiwari A, et al. Complex posterior urethral disruptions: management by combined abdominal transpubic perineal urethroplasty. J Urol 2006;175:1751–4.

32. Koraitim MM. Transpubic urethroplasty revisited: total, superior, or inferior pubectomy. Urology 2010; 75(3):691–4.

33. Terlecki RP, Steele MC, Valadez C, et al. Low yield of early postoperative imaging after anastomotic urethroplasty. Urology 2011;78(2):450–3.

34. Shenfeld OZ, Gdor J, Katz R, et al. Urethroplasty, by perineal approach, for bulbar and membranous urethral strictures in children and adolescents. Urology 2008;71(3):430–3.

35. Cooperberg MR, McAninch JW, Alsikafi NF, et al. Urethral reconstruction for traumatic posterior urethral disruption: outcome of a 25 year experience. J Urol 2007;178:2006–10.

36. Shenfeld OZ, Gofrit ON, Gdor Y, et al. Anastomotic urethroplasty for failed previously treated membranous urethral rupture. Urology 2004;63(5):837–40.

Primary Realignment of Pelvic Fracture Urethral Injuries

Laura Leddy, MD, Bryan Voelzke, MD, Hunter Wessells, MD*

KEYWORDS

• Wounds • Urethra • Urethral stricture • Pelvic fracture

KEY POINTS

- Open primary repair of pelvic fracture urethral injuries (PFUIs) should not be performed due to unacceptably high blood loss and high rates of postoperative erectile dysfunction.
- Primary endoscopic realignment of PFUI is indicated for stable patients with PFUI, especially those with concomitant rectal and/or bladder injury.
- For unstable patients with PFUI, a suprapubic tube should be immediately placed. Endoscopic realignment can then be attempted during the first week after injury provided the patient has been appropriately stabilized.
- Even when primary realignment is successful, the majority of patients will develop a urethral stricture during the first year after the injury.

INTRODUCTION

Pelvic fracture urethral injury (PFUI) is an uncommon yet debilitating consequence of blunt pelvic trauma. The mechanism of these injuries involves major shearing forces at the bulbomembranous junction, resulting in avulsion of the urethra from the fixed urogenital diaphragm.[1] PFUI rates vary from 5% to 25% in small series[2–4]; however, a recent review of the National Trauma Data Bank (NTDB) reported a lower prevalence of 1.54%.[5] The initial management of these devastating injuries involves either primary urethral realignment or suprapubic cystostomy diversion followed by delayed urethroplasty. The potential advantages of primary urethral realignment include an earlier return to voiding, the possibility of avoiding future operative interventions, and better alignment of the proximal/distal urethral segments if an open urethroplasty is necessary in the future.[6,7]

HISTORICAL PERSPECTIVE

PFUI management has changed significantly over the last 80 years. The earliest reported method of operative urethral repair was described by Young in 1929 and involved immediate, primary suturing of the disrupted urethral ends via a perineal approach.[8] This method was abandoned in favor of the retroperitoneal approach because of concerns about placing the injured patient in a dorsal lithotomy position with a concomitant pelvic fracture.[9] Immediate retroperitoneal exploration and primary urethral repair also passed out of favor because of unacceptably high blood loss and high rates of postoperative erectile dysfunction.[4]

Ormond and Cothran first described primary urethral realignment in 1934, by reapproximating the torn urethral ends with a catheter and encouraging re-epithelialization via catheter traction.[10] This technique, referred to as railroading, involved

Department of Urology, Harborview Medical Center, University of Washington School of Medicine, Box 359866, 325 Ninth Avenue, Seattle, WA 98104, USA
* Corresponding author.
E-mail address: wessells@u.washington.edu

Urol Clin N Am 40 (2013) 393–401
http://dx.doi.org/10.1016/j.ucl.2013.04.008
0094-0143/13/$ – see front matter © 2013 Elsevier Inc. All rights reserved.

advancing a catheter across the urethral defect in an antegrade or retrograde fashion to realign the urethra. The catheter remained in place for 4 to 8 weeks. Initially, the patient's catheter was maintained on 500 grams of traction at a 45° angle for the first 5 to 7 days after injury in an effort to realign the proximal and distal urethral ends.[1] The theory supporting use of traction was to provide a scaffold for mucosal regeneration. Increased rates of incontinence were noted following the use of prolonged traction attributed to ischemic damage of the internal sphincter.[11] Canine studies performed in the 1960s also demonstrated that the transected canine posterior urethra did not undergo mucosal re-epithelialization. Instead fibrous tissue filled the intervening gap.[12]

Early techniques for urethral realignment were performed using either Davis interlocking sounds or magnetic sounds.[13] These instruments are of historic interest used in the era before flexible cystoscopy. One sound was placed through the suprapubic tube tract, while the other was passed through the urethra. The sounds were advanced toward each other until the tips either linked together or were brought together via magnetic attraction. The tip of the SP tract sound then followed the penile sound until it exited the urethra, allowing a catheter to be advanced in a retrograde manner into the bladder. An SP tube could be placed for maximal drainage during healing. Primary urethral realignment was the standard of care for treatment of posterior urethral injuries from the 1930s until the 1960s. The technique later fell out of favor because of fear that primary urethral realignment caused further damage to the periprostatic tissue and neurovascular bundles, leading to impaired potency and continence.[1]

In the mid-1950s, Endtner advocated for initial suprapubic cystostomy and no attempt at initial urethral manipulation.[14] This would be followed by delayed, elective repair of the inevitable urethral stricture after 3 to 6 months of suprapubic catheter drainage.[15] Although it generated a nearly 100% stricture rate,[16] this delayed approach was the standard of care for the next 30 years.[1]

Newer techniques pertaining to urethral realignment were introduced in the late 1980s. These techniques evolved into a combination of transurethral and transvesical endourologic procedures in conjunction with fluoroscopy.[1] This technique is postulated to reduce damage to erectile function compared with earlier methods of realignment, because there is no manipulation of the periprostatic tissues and neurovascular bundles.[1]

INDICATIONS

Posterior urethral injury should be considered i male trauma patients who have sustained eithe a pelvic fracture or perineal trauma. Blood at th meatus should increase the level of suspicion Basta and colleagues[17] reported that 92% c male subjects with PFUI had inferomedial pubi bone fractures or pubic symphysis diastasis, an in 88% of subjects, the displacement was greate than 1 cm.

In patients who have sustained blunt trauma t the pelvis or perineum and who are clinically sta ble, a retrograde urethrogram (RUG) should b performed to characterize a potential urethra injury. If a urethral disruption injury is noted, the primary urethral alignment may be indicated. I patients in whom the index of suspicion for urethra injury is high, yet who are clinically unstable, th urologist may attempt placement of a urethra catheter followed by suprapubic catheter if ure thral catheterization is unsuccessful. Retrograd urethrogram for diagnosis and injury staging ca be performed after clinical stabilization of th patient.

Table 1 describes the American Association fc the Surgery of Trauma (AAST) classification fc urethral injuries along with their associated find ings on retrograde urethrogram. In grades 1 an 2, the urethral mucosa is intact, and contras does not extravasate during retrograde urethro gram. In these less severe injury patterns, gentl Foley catheter placement can be performec Grades 3 to 5 injuries range in severity from partia to complete urethral lacerations (**Fig. 1**), and the are amenable to primary urethral realignmer using the techniques outlined in the followin

Table 1		
AAST classification of urethral injuries		
Grade	**Definition**	**Findings on RUG**
1	Contusion	Normal RUG, blood at meatus
2	Stretch injury	Normal RUG, elongation of the urethra
3	Partial disruption	Extravasation of contrast, contrast into bladder
4	Complete disruption	Extravasation of contrast, <2 cm separation, no contrast in bladder
5	Complete disruption	Complete transection, >2 cm urethral separation or injury into prostate or vagina

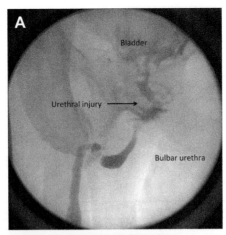

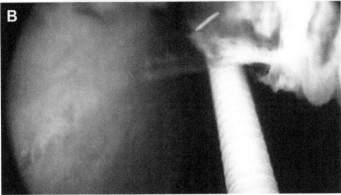

ig. 1. (*A*) Retrograde urethrogram demonstrating partial urethral injury (AAST 3). (*B*) Endoscopic appearance of the lumen with preservation of a portion of the mucosa from 7 to 9 o'clock.

section. Specific indications for primary realignment in hemodynamically stable patients with PFUI include concomitant bladder and bladder neck injury (which makes SP cystostomy difficult or impossible), rectal injury (in which optimized drainage is recommended), and extreme displacement of the bladder and prostate from the membranous urethra (**Fig. 2**). **Fig. 3** outlines the authors' suggested algorithm for the management of PFUI.

TECHNIQUE: RETROGRADE AND ANTEGRADE/RETROGRADE

Primary urethral realignment for posterior urethral injuries can be performed using several techniques. The most commonly described techniques for primary urethral realignment include retrograde and antegrade/retrograde.

Retrograde Approach

A flexible cystoscope is advanced into the urethra to the injured area. In the setting of partial urethral injuries, the cystoscope may be able to navigate

the injury and be advanced directly into the bladder. Otherwise, a glide wire is passed through the damaged portion of the urethra into the bladder. Confirmation that the wire has traversed

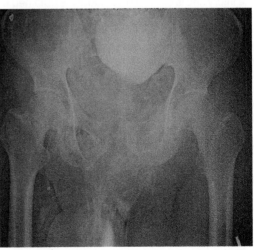

Fig. 2. Cephalad displacement of the urinary bladder by pelvic hematoma in patient with complete urethral disruption (AAST 5).

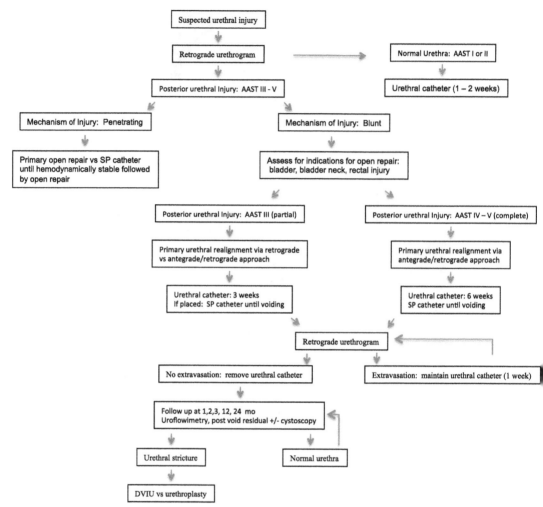

Fig. 3. Algorithm for the management of PFUI.

the injury and is coiled in the bladder is obtained by advancing a 5 F catheter over the wire. The guide wire is then removed leaving the 5 F catheter in place. Urine is then aspirated through the catheter, or, if fluoroscopy is available, a cystogram is performed. After confirmation of the 5 F catheter's position, the guide wire is replaced, and a Council tip catheter is advanced over the wire into the bladder.

Antegrade/Retrograde Approach

This method employs an existing suprapubic tube tract, through which a flexible cystoscope is advanced to the bladder neck. A second cystoscope is advanced retrograde into the urethra. The 2 cystoscopes are advanced toward each other through the damaged portion of the urethra until the light from 1 cystoscope is visible by the other. Fluoroscopic images via a movable C-arm are helpful during this step in severe urethral

disruptions to assess the alignment of the 2 cystoscopes in the anterior/posterior and lateral planes. Once correctly aligned, a wire is advanced through 1 cystoscope into the working port of the other cystoscope, thus establishing access from the suprapubic tract through the injured urethra and out the urethral meatus. The cystoscopes are removed, and a Council tip urethral catheter is passed over the wire across the damaged urethra and into the bladder, where the balloon is inflated. A suprapubic catheter may be left for maximal urinary drainage during healing.

TECHNIQUE: ADDITIONAL CONSIDERATIONS
Timing of Primary Urethral Realignment

Following diagnosis of a partial urethral injury (AAST grade 3), the authors' practice is to make 1 attempt at retrograde urethral catheter placement. If unsuccessful, they proceed with endoscopic alignment via the retrograde approach outlined previously. Primary urethral realignment of a complete injury is often delayed 24 to 72 hours following injury, while the patient is stabilized in the trauma intensive care unit. The bladder is drained with a suprapubic catheter during this time. Delayed primary realignment can take place up to several days after the initial injury in a patient with a suprapubic catheter. The mean and median time to primary realignment in the authors' published series of primary urethral realignment patients was days, with a range of 0 to 7 days.[18]

Placement of a Suprapubic Catheter

In the setting of delayed primary urethral realignment, the patient's bladder is decompressed with a suprapubic catheter. The suprapubic catheter is placed either by the urologist at bedside or under ultrasound guidance in interventional radiology. In pelvic trauma patients, the bladder may be displaced cephalad by significant pelvic hematoma, making ultrasound-guided suprapubic catheter placement a safer option (see **Fig. 2**).

Intraoperative Considerations: Setting, Positioning, Fluoroscopy, Antibiotics

The setting of the primary urethral realignment, at the bedside versus the operating room, is dictated by the stability of the patient and the need for other surgical procedures. To minimize trips to the operating room, the authors' preference is to perform primary urethral realignment in conjunction with other operative procedures, most commonly orthopedic. This provides several benefits, including close hemodynamic monitoring by anesthesia, a sterile environment, timely access to equipment and fluoroscopy, and the ability to perform an open repair of a possible concomitant bladder injury or bladder neck laceration.

The use of flexible cystoscopy allows for the patient to be positioned supine or in dorsal lithotomy position for both the retrograde or antegrade/retrograde approaches. When performed at bedside, the primary realignment is generally performed with the patient supine. Decisions regarding intraoperative positioning can be made with the input of the other surgical services involved in the planned procedures.

Intraoperative fluoroscopy is a helpful adjunct to both retrograde and antegrade/retrograde primary realignment. In the retrograde approach, fluoroscopy can confirm the proximal location of the wire in the bladder. In both approaches, a cystogram can be performed to evaluate for concomitant bladder or bladder neck injury. An intraperitoneal bladder injury or a bladder neck laceration are both indications for open operative repair. During the antegrade/retrograde approach, fluoroscopy can confirm that the 2 cystoscopes are in the appropriate anterior/posterior and lateral plane.

Peri-procedural antibiotic prophylaxis is recommended with either a first-generation cephalosporin or a fluoroquinolone. Practice patterns differ depending on the duration of antibiotic prophylaxis.

Frequency of Technical Success

The reported urethral catheter placement rate via primary realignment is high, ranging from 70 to 93%.[19–22] Other series indicate that if initial primary realignment is unsuccessful, delayed primary realignment in 2 to 3 days may be achievable, as tissue edema may have resolved, enhancing visibility.[20]

Duration of Urethral Catheterizaton

The published duration of urethral catheterization varies from 3 to 6 weeks.[3,4,19–26] The authors' practice is to maintain urethral catheterization for a minimum of 3 weeks for AAST grade 3 injuries and for 6 weeks for complete disruptions (AAST grade 4 and grade 5 injuries).[18] Urethral catheters can be maintained longer if medically necessary as part of the patient's poly-trauma recovery. A peri-catheter retrograde urethrogram or voiding cystourethrogram (VCUG) is performed at the time of catheter removal to confirm absence of urethral extravasation. Bladder drainage should be maintained via urethral catheter or suprapubic catheter until urethral extravasation has fully resolved to reduce the risk of scrotal abscess. If present, the suprapubic catheter can be capped after radiologic confirmation of urethral healing. After confirmation of successful voiding, the suprapubic catheter can be removed.

Surgeon preference dictates whether to leave a suprapubic catheter in addition to the urethral catheter. Orthopedists often prefer removal of a suprapubic catheter after urethral realignment if open reduction and internal fixation are performed for the associated pelvic fracture. If retrograde realignment is achieved, delayed replacement of the SP under controlled conditions may be considered in high-risk patients. If the suprapubic catheter is still present, the authors will cap the SP tube after confirmation of urethral healing and allow voiding per urethra. The SP tube can be removed once the patient is able to successfully void.

Follow-up Protocol

Among patients who failed primary urethral realignment, the mean time to failure was

79 days, with a range of 0 to 288 days.[18] The authors' series indicates that although most patients fail within 6 months of urethral catheter removal, remote failures also occur. Given the high 79% stricture rate noted in their series, the authors' follow-up protocol includes uroflowmetry, postvoid residual and/or cystoscopic evaluation at 1, 2, 3, 12, and 24 months. Patients undergo immediate RUG and/or cystoscopy if symptoms of obstructive voiding manifest. The authors strongly recommend scheduled follow-up after all catheters are removed and do not have patients follow-up on an as-needed basis.

OUTCOMES

Webster and colleagues[27] performed a comprehensive literature review encompassing 538 cases of PFUI dating to the 1950s. The reported stricture rates for patients who underwent primary urethral realignment were 92% versus 100% for delayed open repair. However, it is difficult to interpret these results, as several series in this review used antiquated methods of urethral realignment. Two recent single-institution series comparing primary urethral realignment versus delayed open urethral repair reported stricture rates of 40 to 49% for urethral realignment versus 65% to 100% for open urethral repair (**Table 2**).[6,7]

In the past decade, several single-institution studies of primary urethral realignment were published, reporting urethral stricture rates between 14% and 79% (mean 42%). These rates include patients who have required any additional maneuvers to achieve patency of the urethra, including dilation, direct vision internal urethrotomy, an urethroplasty (see **Table 2**).[6,7,18,20,25,26,28–31]

Of the patients in these single-institution serie who developed a urethral stricture, 78% require endoscopic therapy such as dilation or DVI while 22% went on to require urethroplas (**Table 3**).[6,7,18,20,25,26,28–31] Of note, Olapad Olaopa had patients perform prophylactic urethr dilations and had only 3 patients require urethre plasty.[29] In contrast, the authors' populatic preferred to undergo urethroplasty rather tha multiple endoscopic procedures or repeat inte mittent catheterization.[18]

COMPLICATIONS

Complications that are the direct result of prima urethral realignment are difficult to separate fro the sequelae of the initial traumatic injury. Sever series noted a small rate of complications such a pelvic abscess (2%),[32] urethroscrotal fistu (7%),[33] perineal abscess (16%–25%),[30,34] an septiciemia after delayed primary realigneme (15%).[29] Failure to place a urethral catheter durir primary realignment does not cause addition harm to the patient. In these patients, a suprapub catheter is placed, and delayed urethroplasty performed once urethral stricture develops. The technical success rates of urethral cathete placement are high; yet in 7% to 30% of patient attempts at catheter placement are unsuccessf during primary urethral realignment.[19–22,29]

A common concern in the historic and moder literature is whether endoscopic realignmer makes subsequent urethroplasty more or les difficult. One small series of 7 patients foun

Table 2
Outcomes of modern single-institution series of primary urethral realignement. Stricture rates denote all patients who required additional therapy to achieve urethral patency including dilation, direct vision internal urethrotomy, and urethroplasty

Author/Year Published	Patients in Series	Average Follow-Up (months)	% Stricture	% Incont.	% ED
Leddy et al,[18] 2012	19	25	79	0	21
Sofer et al,[26] 2010	11	52	45	0	55
Olapade-Olaopa et al,[29] 2010	13	36	23	0	0
Hadjizacharia et al,[20] 2008	21	7	14	NR	NR
Healy et al,[28] 2007	8	41	40	0	40
Mouraviev et al,[6] 2005	57	106	49	18	34
Salehipour et al,[30] 2005	25	20	24	0	16
Tazi et al,[31] 2003	36	34	42	0	19
Ku et al,[7] 2002	40	NR	53	16	25
Moudouni et al,[25] 2001	27	83	52	0	15

Abbreviations: ED, erectile dysfunction; Incont., incontinence; NR, not reported.

Table 3
Interventions performed for the management of urethral stricture in the modern, single-institution series of primary urethral realignment

Authors/Year Published	Patients in Series	# with Stricture	# Needing U-Plasty	# Needing DVIU/Dilation	Ongoing CIC
Leddy et al,[18] 2012	19	14	11	3	0
Sofer et al,[26] 2010	11	5	1	4	3
Olapade-Olaopa et al,[29] 2010	13	3	0	2	10
Hadjizacharia et al,[20] 2008	21	3	0	2	0
Healy et al,[28] 2007	8	4	NR	NR	NR
Mouraviev et al,[6] 2005	57	28	14	28	0
Salehipour et al,[30] 2005	25	6	0	6	0
Tazi et al,[31] 2003	36	15	2	13	0
Ku et al,[7] 2002	40	21	NR	NR	NR
Moudouni et al,[25] 2001	27	12	2	12	0

Abbreviation: CIC, clean intermittent catheterization.

that urethroplasty after primary realignment was half as successful as the uninstrumented group (43% vs 85%).[35] This was thought to be the result of inflammation and fibrosis in the periurethral tissues as a result of instrumentation. Other authors have indicated that urethroplasty after primary urtheral realignment was easier and more successful due to appropriate alignment of the proximal and distal urethral ends of the urethra.[7,23] The authors' experience is that urethroplasty after primary realignment is feasible and has good technical success. In their series of 19 patients who underwent primary realignment, 11 underwent posterior urethroplasty. The authors did not note that posterior urethroplasty was more difficult following previous primary urethral realignment. Three patients in their series required operative maneuvers beyond urethral mobilization, including splitting corporal bodies in 2 patients and an inferior pubectomy on 1 patient. One patient required a urethral repair via the abdominoperineal approach; the other patients in the series underwent urethroplasty via a perineal approach. Mean follow-up for these patients is 3.0 years.[18]

Erectile function and urinary continence rates after primary urethral alignment have been reviewed in the urologic literature. In their comprehensive literature review published in 1983, Webster and colleagues[27] reported the rate of erectile dysfunction after urethral realignment was 52% versus 36% after suprapubic cystostomy and delayed open urethral repair. The reported rate of incontinence in this large review was 7% after realignment and 14% after suprapubic cystostomy and delayed open repair. This review demonstrates a high rate of erectile dysfunction in the realignment group versus the suprapubic

cystostomy group. However, a criticism of this review is that the technique for primary urethral realignment was not uniform, as the cohort was from multiple centers (15) and time periods (1961–1983). In addition there was no standardization of realignment technique or subsequent follow-up duration in many of the studies.

Two modern, single-institution series comparing rates of erectile dysfunction after primary urethral alignment versus suprapubic cystostomy followed by delayed open urtheral repair found erectile dysfunction rates of 25% to 34% versus 15% to 42% and urinary incontinence rates of 0% to 18% versus 15% to 26%.[6,7] The reported rate of postrealignment erectile dysfunction is much lower in the modern series, at 25% to 34% versus 52% in Webster's series. These rates were also similar to the rates of erectile dysfunction (15%–42%) found in the suprapubic cystostomy group. The rates of incontinence after primary urethral realignment remain relatively stable in all 3 series, at 0% to 18% versus 7% in Webster's large review.

Recent single institution series report postprimary realignment rates of erectile dysfunction of 0% to 55% and urinary incontinence rates of 0% to 18% (see **Table 2**).[6,7,18,20,25,26,28–31] Data are not available regarding rates of erectile dysfunction before injury and before the primary realignment procedure; therefore, the authors cannot definitively comment on whether the erectile dysfunction is the result of the injury or the subsequent realignment.

LIMITATIONS

Although the published rates of urethral stricture after primary urethral realignment are high, the procedure does save between 21% to 86% of men from subsequent urethral interventions.[6,7,18,20,25,26,28–31] An additional 78% of patients who develop urethral stricture are saved an invasive surgical procedure such as a urethroplasty (see **Table 3**).

The failure rate aside, there are several limitations to primary urethral realignment. Primary urethral realignment can be a time-consuming procedure. The average published time for the retrograde approach is between 5 and 22 minutes.[23,29,36] The authors noted the average time for the antegrade/retrograde approach to be longer at 74 minutes (range 10–284 minutes).[18] Other series have reported the mean time for the antegrade/retrograde approach to be similar, at 40 to 75 minutes (range 30–145 minutes).[25,26]

Primary urethral realignment can be a resource-intense procedure for a several reasons. First, the antegrade/retrograde approach requires additional personnel, as 2 urologists are needed. In addition, close follow-up in the first 3 months after the injury is necessary because of high rates of stricture formation following urethral catheter removal. Lastly, there are issues related to the patient's poly-trauma, such as orthopedic injuries that may delay urological reconstruction if primary realignment fails. In such a circumstance, a suprapubic cathether may need to be reinserted in the operating room or by interventional radiology personnel. In such an instance, the patient will require frequent suprapubic catheter changes until an attempt at minimally invasive therapy or posterior urethroplasty can be made.

Urethral realignment is not indicated for primary treatment of patients with bladder neck or prostatic lacerations caused by pelvic fracture. These particular injuries are surgical emergencies and should be repaired during the index hospitalization once the patient is hemodynamically stable.[37] These patients continue to be managed with immediate open repair because of higher rates of sphincter incompetence or bladder neck contracture if the urothelial defect is not surgically repaired.

SUMMARY

In the past 80 years, debate has been ongoing in the urologic and trauma literature on the safest method of managing PFUI, the method that will result in the highest rates of continence and potency and the lowest rates of stricture formation. This debate has changed from immediate open surgical repair to rudimentary forms of urethral realignment to suprapubic drainage with delayed urethral stricture repair. In the past 30 years,

practice patterns have returned to favor early urethral realignment via endourologic methods. Based on what is available in the urologic literature, combined with the authors' own experience, primary endoscopic urethral realignment following PFUI results in high rates of symptomatic urethral stricture requiring further operative treatment. However, this technique spares a significant number of patients any further urethral intervention and an even greater number of patients the need for a subsequent urethroplasty. Thus, the authors continue to recommend primary urethral realignment after PFUI if it can be performed expediently and without subjecting the patient to additional risks. Close follow-up of these patients remains imperative after initial catheter removal because of cases of delayed stricture formation.

REFERENCES

1. Koraitim MM. Pelvic fracture urethral injuries: the unresolved controversy. J Urol 1999;161(5):1433–41.
2. Pokorny M, Pontes JE, Pierce JM Jr. Urological injuries associated with pelvic trauma. J Urol 1979; 121(4):455–7.
3. Guille F, Cippola B, el Khader K, et al. Early endoscopic realignment for complete traumatic rupture of the posterior urethra—21 patients. Acta Urol Belg 1998;66(2):55–8.
4. Coffield KS, Weems WL. Experience with management of posterior urethral injury associated with pelvic fracture. J Urol 1977;117(6):722–4.
5. Bjurlin MA, Fantus RJ, Mellett MM, et al. Genitourinary injuries in pelvic fracture morbidity and mortality using the National Trauma Data Bank. J Trauma 2009;67(5):1033–9.
6. Mouraviev VB, Coburn M, Santucci RA. The treatment of posterior urethral disruption associated with pelvic fractures: comparative experience of early realignment versus delayed urethroplasty. J Urol 2005;173(3):873–6.
7. Ku J, Kim ME, Jeon YS, et al. Management of bulbous urethral disruption by blunt external trauma: the sooner, the better? Urology 2002; 60(4):579–83.
8. Young HH. Treatment of complete rupture of the posterior urethra, recent or ancient, by anastomosis. J Urol 1929;21:417.
9. Clark SS, Prudencio RF. Lower urinary tract injuries associated with pelvic fractures. Diagnosis and management. Surg Clin North Am 1972;52(1):183–201.
10. Wilkinson FO. Rupture of the posterior urethra with a review of twelve cases. Lancet 1961;1(7187): 1125–9.
11. Turner-Warwick R. Prevention of complications resulting from pelvic fracture urethral injuries—and

from their surgical management. Urol Clin North Am 1989;16(2):335–58.

2. McRoberts JW, Ragde H. The severed canine posterior urethra: a study of two distinct methods of repair. J Urol 1970;104(5):724–9.

3. Porter JR, Takayama TK, Defalco AJ. Traumatic posterior urethral injury and early realignment using magnetic urethral catheters. J Urol 1997;158(2):425–30.

4. Endtner B. Bengt Johanson plastic surgery in treatment of traumatic stricture and rupture of the urethra. Z Unfallmed Berufskr 1958;51(4):302–6.

5. Weems WL. Management of genitourinary injuries in patients with pelvic fractures. Ann Surg 1979;189(6):717–23.

6. Koraitim MM. Pelvic fracture urethral injuries: evaluation of various methods of management. J Urol 1996;156(4):1288–91.

7. Basta AM, Blackmore CC, Wessells H. Predicting urethral injury from pelvic fracture patterns in male patients with blunt trauma. J Urol 2007;177(2):571–5.

8. Leddy LS, Vanni AJ, Wessells H, et al. Outcomes of endoscopic realignment of pelvic fracture associated urethral injuries at a level 1 trauma center. J Urol 2012;188(1):174–8.

9. Follis HW, Koch MO, McDougal WS. Immediate management of prostatomembranous urethral disruptions. J Urol 1992;147(5):1259–62.

10. Hadjizacharia P, Inaba K, Teixeira PG, et al. Evaluation of immediate endoscopic realignment as a treatment modality for traumatic urethral injuries. J Trauma 2008;64(6):1443–9 [discussion: 1449–50].

11. Herschorn S, Thijssen A, Radomski SB. The value of immediate or early catheterization of the traumatized posterior urethra. J Urol 1992;148(5):1428–31.

12. Londergan TA, Gundersen LH, van Every MJ. Early fluoroscopic realignment for traumatic urethral injuries. Urology 1997;49(1):101–3.

13. Gheiler EL, Frontera JR. Immediate primary realignment of prostatomembranous urethral disruptions using endourologic techniques. Urology 1997;49(4):596–9.

14. Jepson BR, Boullier JA, Moore RG, et al. Traumatic posterior urethral injury and early primary endoscopic realignment: evaluation of long-term follow-up. Urology 1999;53(6):1205–10.

25. Moudouni SM, Patard JJ, Manunta A, et al. Early endoscopic realignment of post-traumatic posterior urethral disruption. Urology 2001;57(4):628–32.

26. Sofer M, Mabjeesh NJ, Ben-Chaim J, et al. Long-term results of early endoscopic realignment of complete posterior urethral disruption. J Endourol 2010;24(7):1117–21.

27. Webster GD, Mathes GL, Selli C. Prostatomembranous urethral injuries: a review of the literature and a rational approach to their management. J Urol 1983;130(5):898–902.

28. Healy CE, Leonard DS, Cahill R, et al. Primary endourologic realignment of complete posterior urethral disruption. Ir Med J 2007;100(6):488–9.

29. Olapade-Olaopa EO, Atalabi OM, Adekanye AO, et al. Early endoscopic realignment of traumatic anterior and posterior urethral disruptions under caudal anaesthesia—a 5-year review. Int J Clin Pract 2010;64(1):6–12.

30. Salehipour M, Khezri A, Askari R, et al. Primary realignment of posterior urethral rupture. Urol J 2005;2(4):211–5.

31. Tazi H, Ouali M, Lrhorfi MH, et al. Endoscopic realignment for post-traumatic rupture of posterior urethra. Prog Urol 2003;13(6):1345–50.

32. Patterson DE, Barrett DM, Myers RP, et al. Primary realignment of posterior urethral injuries. J Urol 1983;129(3):513–6.

33. Cohen JK, Berg G, Carl GH, et al. Primary endoscopic realignment following posterior urethral disruption. J Urol 1991;146(6):1548–50.

34. Fowler JW, Watson G, Smith MF, et al. Diagnosis and treatment of posterior urethral injury. Br J Urol 1986;58(2):167–73.

35. Singh BP, Andankar MG, Swain SK, et al. Impact of prior urethral manipulation on outcome of anastomotic urethroplasty for post-traumatic urethral stricture. Urology 2010;75(1):179–82.

36. Kielb SJ, Voeltz ZL, Wolf JS. Evaluation and management of traumatic posterior urethral disruption with flexible cystourethroscopy. J Trauma 2001;50(1):36–40.

37. Mundy AR, Andrich DE. Pelvic fracture-related injuries of the bladder neck and prostate: their nature, cause and management. BJU Int 2010;105(9):1302–8.

Reconstruction of Traumatic and Reoperative Anterior Urethral Strictures via Excisional Techniques

Lee C. Zhao, MD[a], Steven J. Hudak, MD[b], Allen F. Morey, MD[a],*

KEYWORDS

• Urethral stricture • Urethroplasty • Reoperative

KEY POINTS

- Reoperative urethroplasty may be compromised by poor tissue vascularity.
- Excision of poorly vascularized scar is important for successful reconstruction.

Urethroplasty is the gold standard for treatment of anterior urethral strictures. Reported success rates for excisional and primary anastomosis range from 86% to 99%.[1–3] Success rates for substitution urethroplasty are lower, but remain high at 80% to 90%[4–6] for oral mucosal grafts, and 75% to 87%[7,8] for penile skin flaps. For patients with stricture recurrence, reoperative urethroplasty is rendered more challenging by the presence of dense scar tissue and poor tissue vascularity. Further, patients having prior substitution urethroplasty may have a concomitant shortage of donor sites for penile skin flap or oral mucosa graft. For these reasons, our approach to reoperative urethroplasty has centered on an excisional strategy when possible. The role of excisional reoperative urethroplasty is highlighted in this article.

PREOPERATIVE EVALUATION

Nearly all patients with stricture recurrence after urethral reconstruction present with recurrent voiding symptoms. At first, imaging studies including retrograde urethrography (RUG) and voiding cystourethrography (VCUG), when possible, are performed because the radiographic appearance of strictures is known to change dramatically over time after intervention.[9] Patients who have previously undergone urethroplasty, especially substitution techniques, often have irregularities on RUG. Urethroscopy is helpful to determine the caliber of the stricture in such cases; our practical general rule for questionable cases is that, if a 16-French flexible cystoscope can be passed through the area of narrowing, we do not offer surgical repair for those areas. In cases in which the patient has an obliterative stricture and a suprapubic tube has been placed, antegrade urethroscopy may be performed with the flexible cystoscope via the suprapubic tube tract.

Endoscopic management with urethrotomy or balloon dilation is performed if there are short, non-obliterative strictures. If a stricture is not amenable to endoscopic management or has failed previous

Funding: None.
Conflict of Interest: None.
Disclaimer: The opinions expressed in this document are solely those of the authors and do not represent an endorsement by or the views of the United States Air Force, the United States Army, the Department of Defense or the United States Government.

[a] Department of Urology, UT Southwestern Medical Center, Moss Building, 8th Floor, 5323 Harry Hines Boulevard, Dallas, TX 75390-9110, USA; [b] Department of Surgery, Urology Section, San Antonio Military Medical Center, 3851 Roger Brooke Drive, Fort Sam Houston, San Antonio, TX 78234, USA
* Corresponding author. Department of Urology, UT Southwestern Medical Center, Moss Building, 8th Floor, Suite 112, 5323 Harry Hines Boulevard, Dallas, TX 75390-9110.
E-mail address: allen.morey@utsouthwestern.edu

Urol Clin N Am 40 (2013) 403–406
http://dx.doi.org/10.1016/j.ucl.2013.04.011

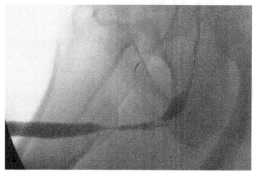

A 53-year-old man with urethral stricture who underwent excision and primary anastomotic urethroplasty.

attempts at endoscopic treatment, reoperative urethral surgical reconstruction is performed.

SURGICAL TECHNIQUE

We attempt to perform reconstruction in a single stage. If more than one stricture is present, we adapt an ascending approach used for primary repair of synchronous strictures.[10] Patient positioning is determined by the location of the stricture (supine for pendulous strictures, adjustable stirrups are used for dorsal lithotomy positioning for bulbar or synchronous strictures requiring concomitant perineal exposure). Serious position-related complications are more common with prolonged time in high lithotomy.[11] If a stricture is present in both the pendulous and bulbar urethra, we repair the pendulous portion first in low lithotomy before raising the legs to minimize time in high lithotomy.

THE CENTRAL ROLE OF EXCISIONAL TECHNIQUES

Scar tissue is poorly vascularized and does not heal normally. Thus, we think that resection of scar

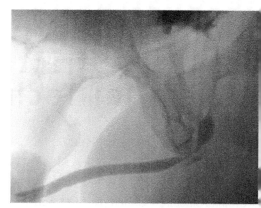

Recurrent stricture treated with urethral stent placed at an outside institution.

tissue is central for the success of urethral reconstruction. When possible, anastomoses should be performed across healthy tissue.

For bulbar strictures, excision and primary anastomosis (EPA) is performed whenever possible. We have found that strictures in the proximal bulbar urethra are especially amenable for this technique.[12] For the patient with posterior urethral stenosis who has previously failed an EPA with us, we usually perform a repeat perineal reconstruction emphasizing proximal exposure via corpora separation; sometimes a combined abdominal perineal approach may be helpful, especially for children or complex cases. The anterior prostatic apex is mobilized off the pubis through the abdominal incision. The urethra is mobilized through the perineal incision. Mobilization through both incisions allows wide proximal exposure and complete scar excision with a tension-free anastomosis. We have found that most patients who have failed initial EPA can be salvaged with repeat EPA.

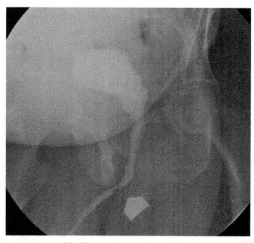

Recurrence of bulbar stricture (*arrow*).

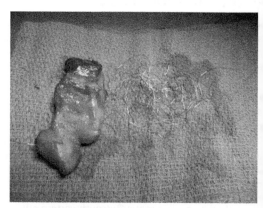

The patient underwent scar excision, removal of UroLume, and repeat urethroplasty.

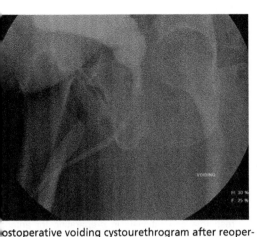

ostoperative voiding cystourethrogram after reoperative excision and primary anastomosis urethroplasty.

UBSTITUTION URETHROPLASTY

When substitution urethroplasty has previously been performed in the bulbar urethra, the type of prior urethroplasty influences the repair. In patients who had a prior ventral onlay graft, we have found that the dorsal aspect of the urethra can be easily dissected from the triangular ligament and corpora cavernosa, thus facilitating straightforward EPA for short recurrences at either ends of the graft. If excessive stricture length precludes EPA, then we prefer to perform an augmented anastomotic urethroplasty with ventral onlay buccal mucosa graft or short penile skin minipatch.[13] In patients who have had a dorsal onlay graft, the dorsal dissection is more difficult because the graft has been quilted to the corporal bodies. However, the abundant ventral bulbar spongiosum facilitates ventral onlay buccal as it normally would in nonreoperative scenarios.

We tend to prefer ventral onlay buccal mucosa graft for longer bulbar strictures because of the ease of exposure and suturing, and the stability of the corpus spongiosum. If there is a poor or absent urethral lumen to graft onto, and the stricture is too long to perform an EPA, overlapping buccal mucosa grafts has proved to be a reliable alternative to multistage reconstruction.[14]

For pendulous strictures, an 18-Fr bougie is placed in the urethra down to the location of the stricture. The urethra is incised ventrally at the midline until normal-caliber urethra is reached. The tissue quality of the urethral plate is examined and stricture length and width assessed. If the width of the urethral plate is at least 8 mm, and there is sufficient healthy non–hair-bearing skin, then we perform a circular fasciocutaneous penile flap.[8] When the dorsal urethral plate is completely diseased, the portion of the dorsal plate containing

the worst scar is excised, the defect is shortened by roof-strip anastomosis if the dorsal defect can be approximated primarily, and a fasciocutaneous penile flap placed ventrally. If the dorsal defect is too long or severe, then a dorsal onlay buccal mucosa graft is placed in conjunction with a ventral fasciocutaneous penile flap.[15] If patients do not have sufficient penile skin for a flap, we perform overlapping buccal mucosa grafts. A short dorsal buccal mucosa graft is placed within the severe defect, and a longer overlapping ventral graft is placed more broadly.[14] When corpus spongiosum is unavailable for ventral graft coverage, tunica dartos, or tunica vaginalis are used, depending on location and tissue availability.

Multistage reconstruction is reserved for patients with long recurrent pendulous strictures who lack sufficient healthy penile skin for flaps, such as those with lichen sclerosus. For these rare cases, the scarred urethra is completely resected and a wide buccal mucosa graft is anastomosed to the proximal and distal end of the normal urethra and secured to the skin edges laterally. Quilting sutures are placed through the graft to fix it to the ventral side of the penis. A bolster dressing is secured with tie-over sutures and left in place for 5 days. The neourethra is then tubularized after approximately 6 months, provided that revision of either anastomosis or augmentation of areas of graft contract is not required.

POSTOPERATIVE FOLLOW-UP

Patients with reoperative stricture are at an increased risk of subsequent stricture recurrence, because the conditions that led to the initial failure (hypospadias, radiation therapy, lichen sclerosis) may still be present. We consequently perform voiding cystourethrogram at the time of catheter removal, and at 6 to 12 months. Patients with voiding symptoms are evaluated with flexible cystoscopy. We define urethroplasty failure as the inability to pass the 16-Fr flexible cystoscope past the obstruction, thus requiring endoscopic treatment or repeat urethroplasty.

SUCCESS OF REOPERATIVE URETHROPLASTY

In a recent University of California, San Francisco, series of 130 patients undergoing reoperative urethroplasty, the investigators reported a success rate of 67% for 1 procedure.[16] Success after 2 procedures was 78% at a median follow-up of 55 months. The investigators performed a variety of repairs: anastomotic, fasciocutaneous penile flap, onlay graft, or combined technique. Anastomotic urethroplasty had lower failure rates

(15%) than other repairs, and was performed nearly half of the time. Longer strictures and complex repairs are more likely to fail. Hypospadias and lichen sclerosis are more likely to result in failure. Most failures occur within 2 years of surgery.

At our institution, we have observed that EPA for reoperative urethroplasty (in well-selected patients) is as successful as EPA performed primarily. Failure after prior substitution repairs can often be treated with EPA. With adequate proximal and distal mobilization, the stricture can be fully excised and an anastomotic repair performed.

SUMMARY

Reoperative urethroplasty is complicated by increased urethral and periurethral scar and the frequent persistence of comorbid conditions that caused the original failure. Nevertheless, by experienced clinicians, reoperative urethral reconstruction can be completed with success rates comparable with those of primary urethroplasty.

REFERENCES

1. Andrich DE, Dunglison N, Greenwell TJ, et al. The long-term results of urethroplasty. J Urol 2003; 170(1):90–2.
2. Barbagli G, de Angelis M, Romano G, et al. Long-term followup of bulbar end-to-end anastomosis: a retrospective analysis of 153 patients in a single center experience. J Urol 2007;178(6):2470–3.
3. Eltahawy EA, Virasoro R, Schlossberg SM, et al. Long-term followup for excision and primary anastomosis for anterior urethral strictures. J Urol 2007; 177(5):1803–6.
4. Heinke T, Gerharz EW, Bonfig R, et al. Ventral onlay urethroplasty using buccal mucosa for complex stricture repair. Urology 2003;61(5):1004–7.
5. Dubey D, Kumar A, Mandhani A, et al. Buccal mucosal urethroplasty: a versatile technique for all urethral segments. BJU Int 2005;95(4):625–9.
6. Elliott SP, Metro MJ, McAninch JW. Long-term followup of the ventrally placed buccal mucosa onlay graft in bulbar urethral reconstruction. J Urol 2003; 169(5):1754–7.
7. Srivastava A, Vashishtha S, Singh UP, et al. Preputial/penile skin flap, as a dorsal onlay or tubularized flap: a versatile substitute for complex anterior urethral stricture. BJU Int 2012;110(11 Pt C):E1101–8.
8. Carney KJ, McAninch JW. Penile circular fasciocutaneous flaps to reconstruct complex anterior urethral strictures. Urol Clin North Am 2002;29(2): 397–409.
9. Terlecki RP, Steele MC, Valadez C, et al. Urethral rest: role and rationale in preparation for anterior urethroplasty. Urology 2011;77(6):1477–81.
10. Langston JP, Robson CH, Rice KR, et al. Synchronous urethral stricture reconstruction via 1-stage ascending approach: rationale and results. J Urol 2009;181(5):2161–5.
11. Anema JG, Morey AF, McAninch JW, et al. Complications related to the high lithotomy position during urethral reconstruction. J Urol 2000;164(2):360–3.
12. Terlecki RP, Steele MC, Valadez C, et al. Grafts are unnecessary for proximal bulbar reconstruction. J Urol 2010;184(6):2395–9.
13. Hudak SJ, Hudson TC, Morey AF. "Minipatch" penile skin graft urethroplasty in the era of buccal mucosa grafting. Arab J Urol 2012;10(4):378–81.
14. Hudak SJ, Lubahn JD, Kulkarni S, et al. Single-stage reconstruction of complex anterior urethral strictures using overlapping dorsal and ventral buccal mucosal grafts. BJU Int 2012;110(4):592–6.
15. Erickson BA, Breyer BN, McAninch JW. Single-stage segmental urethral replacement using combined ventral onlay fasciocutaneous flap with dorsal onlay buccal grafting for long segment strictures. BJU Int 2012;109(9):1392–6.
16. Blaschko SD, McAninch JW, Myers JB, et al. Repeat urethroplasty after failed urethral reconstruction: outcome analysis of 130 patients. J Urol 2012; 188(6):2260–4.

Reconstruction of Radiation-Induced Injuries of the Lower Urinary Tract

Nathaniel K. Ballek, MD*,
Christopher M. Gonzalez, MD, MBA

KEYWORDS

• Radiation • Urethra • Stricture • Bladder neck contracture • Brachytherapy • Urethroplasty

KEY POINTS

• Radiation therapy for prostate cancer has been used with increased frequency in the past 2 decades. Higher radiation doses with modern techniques seem to be a significant risk factor for formation of urethral stricture, bladder neck contracture, and rectourethral fistula.
• Radiation delivered to the apex of the prostate during interstitial therapy is a significant risk factor for the formation of urethral stricture in the bulbar and membranous urethra. Dose modifications may limit formation of urethral stricture.
• Intensity-modulated radiation therapy has shown no increased risk of lower urinary tract injury compared with three-dimensional conformal external beam radiation therapy.
• Urethral stricture caused by radiation therapy is often located in the bulbar and membranous region. Most of these strictures are short, and most often can be repaired with excision and primary anastomosis. Longer strictures are amenable to substitution urethroplasty.
• Rectourethral fistula caused by radiation therapy is a serious complication. Urinary and bowel function can be successfully restored with reconstruction in many patients.

INTRODUCTION

Radiation therapy for the treatment of prostate cancer has been evolving since its introduction in the early twentieth century. The discovery of radioactivity, the weak form of uranium, by Henri Becquerel in 1896 and the discovery of radium by Marie and Pierre Curie in 1898 ushered in a new era in medical technologies.[1] Early knowledge of the effects of radiation on human tissue was identified through incidental exposures by early researchers. The subsequent medical applications with this new technology attempted to maximize the dose of radiation and minimize the effects on normal tissue. The following 2 decades led to refined technologies and techniques of administration to prostate tissue through mainly intracavitary means that were used by prominent urologists of the era, including Hugh Hampton Young.[2] Benjamin Barringer is credited with pioneering the interstitial implantation techniques currently used via a perineal and suprapubic approach using glass-encapsulated radon.[3] The 1930s saw the first use of external beam radiation therapy (EBRT). More effective use of external and interstitial therapies now relies on modern imaging techniques of computed tomography (CT) scans and transrectal ultrasound to maximize treatment and limit side effects.[4]

Prostate cancer is the most common non–skin-related malignancy of men in the United States. In 2012, an estimated 241,740 new cases

Department of Urology, Northwestern University Feinberg School of Medicine, 303 East Chicago Avenue, Tarry 16-703, Chicago, IL 60611, USA
* Corresponding author.
E-mail address: nkballek@gmail.com

Urol Clin N Am 40 (2013) 407–419
http://dx.doi.org/10.1016/j.ucl.2013.04.009
0094-0143/13/$ – see front matter © 2013 Elsevier Inc. All rights reserved.

will be diagnosed, which accounts for 29% of all new cancer diagnoses in men.[5] According to the 2007 American Urological Association guidelines, use of either brachytherapy (BT) or EBRT may be used alone or in combination for first-line therapy for localized prostate cancer.[6] Analysis of the CaPSURE (Cancer of the Prostate Strategic Urologic Research Endeavor) database, a national disease registry of more than 10,000 men, found that radiation therapy was used in more than 20% of newly diagnosed low-risk prostate cancer from 1993 to 2001.[7] This same study also showed an increase in the use of BT from 4% to 22% during the study time period. The SEER (Surveillance, Epidemiology, and End Results) database, which includes primarily men more than the 65 years of age, has shown a rapid adoption of use in recent years of intensity-modulated radiation therapy (IMRT), a modality of EBRT that can deliver high doses of radiation. The use of IMRT compared with three-dimensional conformal EBRT increased from 0.15% of total men treated with EBRT in 2000 to 95.6% in 2008.[8] Despite little knowledge of the long-term genitourinary morbidity, rapid adoption of high-dose IMRT and BT have become more prevalent in the treatment of prostate cancer.

Lower urinary tract injury caused by radiation treatment of pelvic malignancy includes formation of urethral stricture, bladder neck contracture (BNC), and rectourethral fistula (RUF). Each of these conditions can be a serious complication to the patient both physically and mentally. This article focuses on the pathophysiology, risk, evaluation, surgical reconstruction, and long-term considerations for patients with lower urinary tract injury caused by radiation therapy.

PATHOPHYSIOLOGY AND RISK FACTORS FOR LOWER URINARY TRACT INJURY

Radiation interacts with living cells in several ways that make it an effective cancer treatment. The effects may be divided into direct or indirect interactions with ionizing radiation. The direct interaction occurs when the energy from the photon directly damages either the cellular DNA and/or tissue protein. This damage leads to immediate cell death or mutation of the DNA. The indirect interaction occurs when the ionizing radiation interacts with water in the cell and leads to the formation of free radicals that interact with enzymes leading to cell death or future mutation. Both of these interactions lead to cellular injury that can cause division delay, reproductive failure, or interphase death through the apoptosis mechanism, which is more common in rapidly dividing cells.[9] These interactions and resultant cellular injury are dose

dependent and occur in a linear threshold mode When normal tissue is damaged with exposur greater than the injury threshold, several change occur that result in a cycle of scar and subsequer healing. Damage to basement membranes vessels can lead to occlusion, thrombosis, an eventually reduced neovascularization.[10] The sub sequent fibrosis is caused by an increase of fibro blasts that no longer make mature collagen, whic accounts for the atrophy and contraction of th tissue.[11]

Urethral stricture results from replacement of th corpus spongiosum with fibrosis and resultar occlusion of the urethral lumen.[12] With a more thor ough understanding of radiation biology it is logica that increases in radiation doses would result in higher rate of urethral stricture. High-dose-rate B (HDRBT) and EBRT, either alone or in combinatior have been used to achieve higher disease-free sur vival for the treatment of prostate cancer.[4,13–1] This strategy has developed out of improved tech nology and imaging techniques that allow mor focused concentration of radiation to the intende tissue. Data from the CaPSURE database showe the stricture rate for BT to be 1.8%, EBRT 1.7% and combined therapy 5.2%.[17] Another mor recent study compared the rate of stricture forma tion in 1903 patients after EBRT, low-dose-rate BT and HDRBT. The rates of urethral stricture forma tion were 2%, 4%, and 11% respectively, indi cating that despite modern imaging technique and modifications the amount of radiation damag delivered to normal tissue is significant.[18]

The use of HDRBT has shown a high incidenc of urethral stricture formation. Sullivan and col leagues[19] showed that after HDRBT the actuaria rate of urethral stricture formation at 6 years wa estimated to be 12% for all urethral locations an 10.8% for the bulbomembranous location. Overall the investigators concluded that 90% of urethra strictures following HDRBT occur in the bulbo membranous region. When combined with EBRT HDRBT has a similar rate of stricture formatio as HDRBT alone at 11.8%.[14]

As expected, the dose of radiation delivered t the urethra has been shown to be a significant risl factor in the development of urethral stricture a well as the location of the delivered radiatior dosage. Merrick and colleagues[20] has shown that in patients with urethral stricture formation following BT, the dose delivered to the apex of the prostate was significantly higher than in case-controlled pa tients who did not form urethral strictures. By limiting the dosage to the apex of the prostate, the investigators showed a relative risk reduction o stricture formation of greater than 30% Earley and colleagues[21] found that the radiation delivered by w-dose-rate BT within 5 mm of the urethra at the pex of the prostate was significant. Of the patients eated in this study, the 6.5% who formed urethral ricture had roughly 30% more dosage delivered the apex of the prostate.

The amount of radiation delivered per treatment so affects the rate of urethral stricture following eatment. When 18 to 20 Gy of radiation were elivered by HDRBT over 2, 3, or 4 fractionated osages, the stricture rate was different. The fracionated dosages were delivered during a single ospital admission with at least 6 hours between eatments. The urethral stricture rate increased 31.6% when delivered over 2 treatments, ompared with 3.4% for 3 treatments and 2.3% or 4 treatments. The investigators concluded that e amount delivered per treatment was the most gnificant factor in urethral stricture formation, hich led to a change in their treatment algorithm.[22]

EBRT may be delivered in a variety ways. The ost common modern techniques are three-imensional conformal therapy and IMRT, which ave a similarly low rate of stricture formation, typi-ally reported to be less than 3%.[17,18,23] However en who have undergone previous transurethral esection of the prostate before conformal EBRT ave an increased risk of urethral stricture forma-on ranging from 4% to 16%.[24,25] Another high-sk group for urethral stricture formation includes en who undergo adjuvant EBRT therapy for igh-risk prostate cancer following radical prosta-ectomy in whom the rate of urethral stricture for-ation is reported to be as high as 17%.[26]

Proton beam therapy (PBT) uses high-velocity articles instead of photons to deliver energy to e prostate. In theory, PBT delivers less energy normal tissue because the proton's energy is issipated at preset depths depending on the elocity of the proton.[27] Genitourinary complica-ons seem to be comparable with external beam erapies, although limited data make these rates ifficult to compare. In one phase III clinical trial at compared high-dose EBRT alone or with an dditional boost of conformal PBT, the rate of rethral stricture increased from 8% of 99 patients vho received EBRT therapy alone to 19% of 103 atients who received a PBT boost to EBRT.[28]

Data on the rate of formation of BNC after radi-tion are limited; however, it is estimated to be etween 2% and 12%.[17,29-31] The risk factors for e development of BNC following radiation have ot been studied as extensively as urethral stric-ure formation, but it can be inferred that similar actors such as the dose and location of radiation elivery play a major role.

RUF formation following radiation therapy has een reported with greater frequency in the literature over the last decade. The process that re-sults in RUF formation following radiation is specu-lated to be the result of fibrosis and microvascular injury leading to mucosal ulcers and eventual fistu-lization. Lane and colleagues[32] concluded that, before 1997, radiation therapy accounted for only 12% of the total RUF. After 1997, RUF caused by radiation increased to 49.6% of the total RUF re-ported in the literature. The investigators concluded that reporting bias may have been partially respon-sible for this finding but likely the increase in use of radiation therapy for prostate cancer was also responsible. Nonetheless, the overall incidence of RUF is uncommon after EBRT (0%–0.6%)[33,34] and after BT (0.3%–3%).[30,35-37] As with radiation-induced urethral stricture, this process seems to be dose dependent, but this has not been confirmed.

The risk of RUF may increase after endoscopic or open manipulation of the urethra, prostate, or rectum following radiation therapy. In one study, RUF was linked to postradiation transurethral resection of the prostate in 38%, postradiation rectal biopsy in 38%, and argon beam therapy for postradiation proctitis in 13% of patients.[38] This same study also showed a high rate of concomitant urethral and rectal strictures, which may cause high-pressure elimination, a contributing factor in the development of RUF.

Salvage therapy after primary radiotherapy for recurrent prostate cancer significantly increases genitourinary complications. Salvage radical pros-tatectomy can result in an anastomotic urethral stricture rate of up to 41%[39,40] with an average rate of 20%.[41] Salvage cryotherapy results in ure-thral sloughing and subsequent stricture formation in 15% of patients,[42,43] BNC in up to 28% of patients,[43,44] and RUF in 3.4% of patients.[45,46] Salvage BT after primary radiotherapy results in grade 3 to 4 genitourinary toxicity in 14% to 47% of patients,[47,48] but specific percentages of urethral stricture are difficult to determine. Following salvage BT, RUF has been reported to occur in up to 12% of patients.[41,49] High-intensity focused ultrasound (HIFU), when used for biochemical recurrence following radiation therapy, results in BNC formation in 17% of patients and RUF formation in up to 16% of cases.[41]

PATIENT EVALUATION

Multiple urinary symptoms may occur as a result of radiation injury to the lower urinary tract. Storage-related symptoms such as frequency, urgency, and urge-related incontinency occur mainly as a result of bladder damage and loss of capacity; postmicturition and obstructive symptoms such as hesitancy, postvoid dribbling, and weakened stream occur mostly secondary to occlusion of the lower urinary tract. Up to 70% of patients may report these symptoms in a progressive manner that may even manifests months or years after the initial radiation injury.[12] A validated questionnaire specific to urethral strictures has not been fully established; however, Jackson and colleagues[50] provided methodology and initial results for a urethral stricture–specific questionnaire with good content and criterion validity to assess urinary complaints. When fully developed, such a tool may aid in the noninvasive evaluation and follow-up for patients with urethral stricture disease. Urinary tract infection, hematuria, or acute urinary retention may also occur in these patients, but less commonly as the presenting complaint. Physical examination can be used to determine urethral meatus patency and may reveal suprapubic fullness if urinary obstruction is present. On rectal examination, a RUF may be palpated, especially if the defect is large.

Diagnostic studies useful for the evaluation of urethral strictures and BNC consist of urinary flow studies, urodynamics, endoscopic studies, and radiologic evaluation. Urinary flow studies are commonly performed and often show a flat curve with low urinary flow rate in men with obstruction from BNC or urethral stricture disease.[51] Urodynamic studies may be helpful to determine whether a patient is a candidate for reconstructive repair of BNC following radiation therapy, although catheter placement may be challenging. For patients with bladder volumes less than 200 mL or severe detrusor instability, conservative measures to increase bladder volume may be attempted before reconstruction. However, other options such as bladder augmentation before reconstruction or urinary diversion can be discussed with the patient.[52,53] Postvoid residual may also be performed but this study is nonspecific and may be subject to user variation.[54] Retrograde urethrography offers the ability to determine the length and location of the obstruction (**Figs. 1** and **2**). If necessary, voiding cystourethrogram allows for full evaluation of the posterior urethra as well as the urethra proximal to the stricture if retrograde urethrogram is inconclusive.[12] If a suprapubic tube is present, simultaneous antegrade endoscopy and retrograde urethrography can be performed (**Fig. 3**). MRI and CT scan rarely provide useful staging information before urethroplasty. Ultrasound of the urethral stricture may also provide useful staging information about the extent of the spongiofibrosis.[55]

RUF is often more obvious than urethral stricture or BNC and presents with urine persistently leaking from the rectum. The fistula typically develops

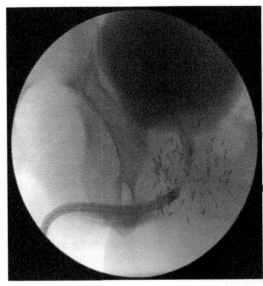

Fig. 1. A stricture involving the bulbar and membranous urethra following BT.

several months to years after treatment with radiation. In addition to the urinary leakage, patients may present with pneumaturia, dysuria, perineal pain, or pelvic pain. Fecaluria is less common with RUF than colovesical fistula because of the higher pressure of the urethra compared with the bowel.[56] Digital rectal examination may assist with the diagnosis if the defect is large. Retrograde urethrogram and cystogram should be performed to confirm the suspected diagnosis and to determine whether there is a concomitant urethral

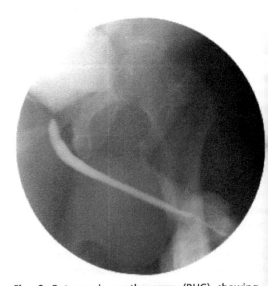

Fig. 2. Retrograde urethrogram (RUG) showing radiation-induced BNC following radical prostatectomy and adjuvant EBRT.

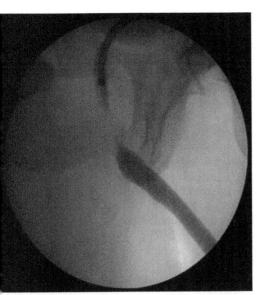

Fig. 3. Combined antegrade endoscopy and RUG to delineate the extent of a radiation-induced urethral stricture.

stricture or BNC in addition to the RUF (**Fig. 4**). Proctoscopy and cystoscopy should also be performed under anesthesia to fully delineate the location and extent of the fistula and guide planning. Examination should also focus on evaluation of a rectal stricture, because almost all patients who are treated with BT have some degree of rectal stenosis.[57] Biopsy should be taken of all fistula tracts before surgery to assess for cancer recurrence at the fistula site. Abdominal and pelvic imaging with CT or magnetic resonance imaging

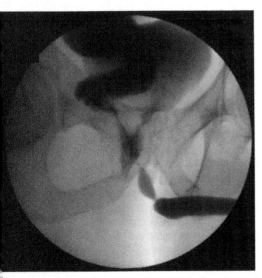

Fig. 4. RUG showing a rectourethral fistula and concomitant urethral stricture.

also helps to delineate the location of the fistula and the degree of surrounding tissue viability.[32]

Diversion with a colostomy or ileostomy has been reported before or at the time of definitive reconstructive management for tissue healing and symptomatic improvement.[32,38,58,59] Although it has been stated that all patients who develop a complex RUF following radiation therapy should undergo fecal diversion, this has not been established.[60] Mundy and Andrich[56] reported a series of radiation-induced RUF repaired with and without fecal diversion. The investigators showed no impact of preoperative fecal diversion on the success of the repair. It was postulated by the investigators that, if fecal diversion was not performed after the initial diagnosis, then a colostomy was not necessary at the time of repair. In general, the decision to perform fecal diversion should be based on the viability of the tissue surrounding the RUF.[61] Counseling is important with these patients because urinary and fecal diversion can be used as definitive long-term management in lieu of reconstruction for symptomatic relief.[38,58] Permanent fecal diversion may be considered in patients with extensive damage to the rectum and anal sphincter with a low probability of fecal continence after surgery.

When considering reconstruction of the urinary tract for RUF, urodynamic studies should be considered. Urodynamics may be difficult to obtain in patients with RUF, because the bladder may not hold adequate volumes because of urinary leakage. Nonetheless an assessment of bladder capacity is necessary. As with patients diagnosed with radiation-induced urethral stricture or BNC, men with a radiation-induced RUF and a significantly limited bladder capacity are often best suited for urinary diversion with cystectomy and ileal conduit.

Sexual function should be evaluated and assessed before and following reconstruction of lower urinary tract injuries caused by radiation. Sexual function, as assessed by patient report, was preserved in the 50% of patients undergoing anterior urethroplasty for radiation-induced urethral stricture who reported normal sexual function before surgery. However, validated patient-reported outcome measures were not used in this study.[62] The International Index of Erectile Function (IIEF) questionnaire has been helpful in the assessment of men with urethral stricture of various causes. Erickson and colleagues[63] reported on a prospective analysis of 52 men who underwent urethroplasty for anterior urethral stricture disease. Thirty-eight percent (20/52) of patients experienced worsened erectile function after surgery. At 6 months following urethroplasty, 90% (18/20) of these men recovered their preoperative level of sexual function. Ejaculatory function also seems to be preserved following urethroplasty for anterior urethral stricture disease of various causes. Prospective use of the Male Sexual Health Questionnaire has shown that 89% (38/43) of men report stable or improved ejaculatory function after surgery.[64] Ejaculatory function has not been evaluated in men with radiation-induced urethral stricture diseases. Doppler ultrasound may prove useful to assess penile blood flow before urethroplasty for stricture disease, but its usefulness to assess erectile function in patients with radiation injury to the lower urinary tract remains unknown. The impact of lower urinary tract reconstruction on sexual function in men with radiation-induced BNC or RUF remains to be studied.

URETHRAL STRICTURE SURGICAL RECONSTRUCTION

Dilation and endoscopic incision of urethral stricture caused by radiation is often reported with high success in the radiation oncology literature, although there is a paucity of data on long-term follow-up and recurrence following these endoscopic options.[19,20,65] A limited number of studies have specifically addressed outcomes following urethroplasty in men with urethral stricture formation after radiation therapy.

The first report on reconstructive outcomes in men with radiation-induced urethral stricture disease focused on a small single-center series that showed that excision and primary anastomosis (EPA) was effective for strictures less than 2 cm in 6 of 7 patients. One patient who underwent a genital skin fasciocutaneous flap for a stricture less than 2 cm recurred. Time to recurrence, incontinence, and sexual function outcomes were not reported in this study.[66]

A retrospective, multiinstitutional study reported on the follow-up of 30 patients who underwent reconstructive repair of urethral strictures following radiation therapy for prostate cancer. The study population consisted of 15 men (50%) treated with EBRT alone, 7 men (24%) treated with BT alone, and 8 patients (26%) treated with combined EBRT and BT. All of the urethral strictures were in the bulbomembranous urethra, averaging 2.9 cm in length with a range of 1.5 cm to 7 cm. EPA was used in 24/30 (80%) patients with an average stricture length of 3 cm. The remaining repairs consisted of genital fasciocutaneous skin flap use in 4/30 (13%) and buccal graft onlay in 2/10 (7%) patients, with an average stricture length of 4.3 cm. A total of 27% (9/30) of the patients in this series recurred at a mean of 5.1 months and 2 required balloon dilation. No patients required eventual urinary diversion. The new onset of

incontinence was seen in 50% (15/30) of men and resolved in 3/30 (10%). An artificial urinar sphincter (AUS) was placed in 4/30 (13%) men Erectile function was preserved in the men who reported normal preoperative function.[62]

In the largest reported single series to date, Glas and colleagues[67] retrospectively reported on total of 29 men with urethral stricture formatio following radiation treatment of prostate cancer Eleven patients treated with EBRT alone (38% were included; radical prostatectomy followed b adjuvant EBRT, 7 (24%); combined EBRT/BT in (24%); and BT alone 4 (14%). The average strictur length was 2.6 cm in the series, with location iden tified in the bulbar urethra, 12/29 (41%); membra nous urethra, 12/29 (41%); bladder neck, 3/2 (10%); and panurethral, 2/29 (7%). EPA was per formed in 22/29 (76%) patients, whereas 5/2 (17%) underwent substitution urethroplasty with buccal graft, and 2/29 (7%) with fasciocutaneou flap onlay. One EPA, 1 buccal graft, and 1 fasciocu taneous flap onlay case each recurred for an overal series success rate of approximately 90%. The new onset of urinary incontinence was reported in only 2 patients (7%) with 1 patient opting for an AUS to manage urinary incontinence. Erectile functior was not reported before or after surgery.

Although limited in patient number and design these studies show acceptable success rate with EPA in patients undergoing urethroplasty for short proximally located, radiation-induced urethra strictures. Substitution urethroplasty seems to be most effective for anatomically more distal stric tures in the bulbar or penile urethral and those o greater length. Longer follow-up is needed to assess the durability of these outcomes.

The technical approach for radiation-induced urethral stricture disease is similar to that for other causes. For proximally located stricture disease the patient may be placed in the exaggerated o dorsal lithotomy position for perineal exposure o the urethra to the level of the prostate. Mobilizatior of the urethra off the corpora cavernosa to the proximal penile urethra is often necessary to achieve a tension-free anastomosis. Other exten sive maneuvers such as splitting the corpora cav ernosa or removal of the pubic bone have beer described but are rarely necessary.[68]

Complete scar excision to the level of the pros tatic apex is often necessary in patients with bul bomembranous stricture disease. At times, the ability to place sutures in the apex of the prostate for a primary anastomosis with the bulbar urethra may be limited with standard needle drivers. Use of the Capio device (Boston Scientific) can assis in placing these proximal sutures at the desired depth (**Fig. 5**). The device was originally designec

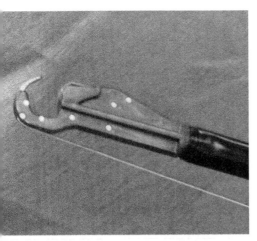

Fig. 5. The Capio device with a preloaded suture.

for placement of sutures in complex female urology procedures. The curve of the Capio device makes it ideal for passing suture at an oblique angle, and is superior to other suture-passing devices used in laparoscopy that only pass suture at a right angle. With these maneuvers it is possible to properly place sutures into the mucosa of the apical prostate to create a watertight anastomosis with the bulbar urethra.

BLADDER NECK RECONSTRUCTION

BNC after radiation therapy has unique considerations of management compared with BNC following radical prostatectomy. The patients undergoing radiation therapy who develop BNC often cannot tolerate a suprapubic tube and are at high risk of bladder instability as well as low bladder capacity.[53] There are limited data on outcomes following open reconstruction for recalcitrant BNC in men with a history of radiation for treatment of prostate cancer. The reconstructive approaches and outcomes following BNC of various causes, including radiation therapy, are summarized in **Table 1**. For bladder neck reconstruction following primary radiation therapy for prostate cancer, salvage prostatectomy (SP) can be considered for reconstructive therapy following failure of endoscopic management. Mundy and Andrich[53] reported on 9 patients undergoing SP for BNC that resulted in 3 patients developing recurrent BNC and 1 patient requiring an AUS for management of incontinence. For patients undergoing open SP for biochemical recurrence after radiation therapy, the de novo BNC formation rate was 41% following surgery in one large single-center study.[40] Robotic SP is also feasible and may have less morbidity than open SP with a BNC incidence of 9%.[69]

Almost all patients in both the open and robotic SP series developed some degree of urinary incontinence, with only 30% regaining continence at 3 years in the open SP series.[40,69] In men with preoperative sexual potency, approximately 30% remained potent in both the open SP and the robotic SP series.[40,69]

In the setting of a recalcitrant BNC following radical prostatectomy with adjuvant EBRT, the reconstruction of a patent vesicourethral anastomosis may involve a combined abdominoperineal, abdominal, or a perineal approach. Reconstructive surgery is best considered only after multiple failed attempts at endoscopic management including cold or hot knife incision, laser ablation, dilation, limited transurethral resection, or failed urethral stent placement. Early reports of open reconstruction involved a combined abdominoperineal approach that used pubectomy, and the use of omentum or rectus muscle to support a primary anastomosis or a penile fasciocutaneous flap for onlay over the stricturotomy.[70,71] Subsequent larger series described reconstruction using a combined open abdominal or perineal approach along with endoscopic techniques to reduce overall operative time and morbidity.[72,73] Outcomes in these series were variable and no standardization of approach for these patients has been established.

In those men with a lengthy BNC following radical prostatectomy and radiation, an abdominoperineal approach is an effective reconstructive option. Often a transpubic approach is performed to access the stenosed section of the bladder neck and membranous urethra. A perineal approach is used to obtain access to the bulbar urethra for mobilization and eventual anastomosis. The primary advantage of this combined approach includes the ability to excise all diseased tissue to create a tension-free primary anastomosis in an irradiated field compared with a perineal or transpubic approach alone (**Fig. 6**).

A transpubic approach can be used for limited BNC to preserve the urethral sphincter and continence. Complete or partial pubectomy is performed to obtain access to the bladder neck with limited mobilization of the urethra and bladder to avoid extensive tissue damage or rectal injury in the radiated field. In the author's experience, the use of an anterior bladder wall advancement flap has proved successful to augment BNC of up to 3 cm (**Fig. 7**). Pfalzgraf and colleagues[72] reported a series of 20 men treated for BNC after prostatectomy with an intact external urethral sphincter. A retropubic approach and use of a Grunewald retractor to assist in the placement of anastomotic sutures for a primary anastomosis was used in all patients. An initial patency rate of 60% was

Table 1
Outcomes of reconstruction for recalcitrant BNC

Study	# Patients	Approach	Cause (N)	Tissue Interposition (N)	Patency (%)	Postoperative Urinary Incontinence (%)
Schlossberg et al,[70] 1995	2	Abdominoperineal	RRP (2)	Omental flap (2)	100	0
Wessells et al,[71] 1998	4	Abdominoperineal (1) Transpubic (2) Perineal (1)	RRP (1) SP (1) RPP (2)	Omental flap (1) Penile skin flap (1) Rectus flap (1)	100	100
Mundy et al,[53] 2012	9	Retropubic SP (9)	EBRT±BT (9)	0	66	11
Pfalzgraf et al,[72] 2011	20	Retropubic (VUA)	RRP (20)	0	60	33
Simonato et al,[73] 2012	11	Perineal (VUA)	LRP (3) RRP (8)	0	100	94

Abbreviations: LRP, laparoscopic radical prostatectomy; RRP, radical retropubic prostatectomy; SP, salvage prostatectom
VUA, vesicourethral anastomosis.

achieved, with additional endoscopic resection increasing the patency rate to 95%. Urinary incontinence was reported at 33% following successful repair.

RECTOURETHRAL FISTULA REPAIR

Postsurgical RUF in the absence of radiation therapy is rare, with an incidence of less than 1% after radical prostatectomy.[74] If surgical repair is warranted after a trial of conservative therapy, less invasive approaches may be used, such as transanal or transanosphincteric approach, wit success rates approaching 100%. These opera tions are performed in the prone position with pr mary closure of the prostatic and rectal defect a well as mucosal advancement flaps.[60,75,76] I contrast, radiation-induced RUF mostly does no respond to conservative methods and more ofte requires reconstruction and tissue interpositio for successful resolution.[77] Urethral stricture an BNC are present concomitantly in 28% of patient

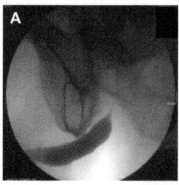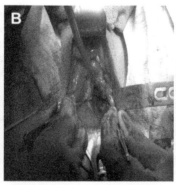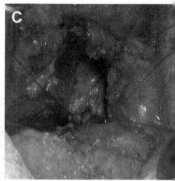

Fig. 6. (*A*) RUG of lengthy BNC after radical prostatectomy and adjuvant EBRT. (*B*) Perineal approach to mobiliz the urethra. (*C*) Transpubic approach to resect contracture and complete the anastomosis of the bulbar urethr and bladder neck.

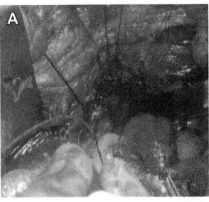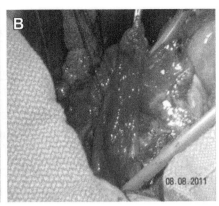

Fig. 7. (*A*) Urethrotomy of a BNC. (*B*) Anterior bladder wall advancement flap for closure of the urethrotomy.

with RUF following radiation therapy, which further complicates surgical repair in this cohort.[59]

Approaches for the repair of radiation-induced RUF consist of transanal, transanosphincteric, transperineal, and abdominal techniques. In the setting of a radiation-induced RUF, reconstructive considerations include initial fecal and urinary diversion, adequate exposure of the fistula, the use of well-vascularized tissue for interposition, and repair of concomitant disorders of the urethra and rectum. The likelihood of success is subject to the experience of the surgeon(s) involved. Large studies specifically addressing approaches and outcomes after reconstruction for radiation-induced RUF formation are limited in number, with some outcome variables not fully available (**Table 2**).

Less invasive techniques more commonly used for uncomplicated RUF have limitations that make repairs with this approach technically difficult or inadequate for radiation-induced RUF. A transanal approach is discouraged for radiation-induced RUF repair because of limited exposure and inability to access the lower urinary tract other than the prostate for repair. A transanosphincteric (York-Mason) approach allows for better exposure of the RUF with limited permanent damage to the anal sphincter. This approach also provides adequate space for the use of tissue interposition with gracilis muscle flaps, rectal advancement flaps, and multilayered closure. However, similar to the transanal approach, larger or complex defects are challenging with the transanosphincteric approach, because strictures of the bulbar and membranous urethra often cannot be fully exposed and repaired.[59]

The transperineal approach is most commonly used for management of large, complex RUF associated with radiation treatment.[56,59,66,78] Advantages of this approach include wide exposure for large fistulae and the ability to address concomitant disorders of the rectum and urethra. Tissue interposition for large defects of the urethra can be performed adequately with graft of flap, and the ability to interpose gracilis flaps is readily available. Small rectal defects can be repaired directly with primary closure. An abdominoperineal resection with staged coloanal anastomosis can be used if the tissue of the rectum is not adequate for primary closure or a rectal stricture is present.[32]

An abdominal approach is not commonly used, but it can be used in the setting of a RUF after radiation therapy that necessitates SP in the same setting as repair. This approach does not allow access to the anterior urethra or distal rectum, which necessitates perineal exposure for concomitant anterior urethral stricture or RUF not located in the prostatic urethra. The use of omentum and peritoneum can be used with this approach to interpose this tissue between the rectal repair and vesicourethral anastomosis.[56]

Long-term quality of life (QOL) and functional outcome of the fecal and urinary systems after complex RUF repair have only recently been addressed in the literature. Samplaski and colleagues[79] presented the results of 12 patients who completed symptom-specific QOL questionnaires concerning urinary and fecal outcome following successful transperineal repair of a complex RUF repair with gracilis muscle interposition. RUF cause was radical prostatectomy in 4 (33%), BT alone in 3 (25%), combined EBRT and BT in 3 (25%), cryoablation in 1 (~8%), cryoablation and EBRT in 1 (~8%), and imperforate anus in 1 (~8%) The fecal function impact on patient QOL was generally better than urinary function. Only 4 of 12 (25%) patients who had fecal incontinence were managed with adult diapers and did not report significant social embarrassment. In contrast, 9 of 12 (75%) patients reported some degree of urinary incontinence, with 4 (33%) having significant stress-related incontinence and 4 (33%) having significant urge-related incontinence. Only 2

Table 2
Outcomes after reconstruction for RUF following radiation therapy

Study	# Patients	Approach (N)	Cause (N)	Tissue Interposition (N)	Recurrence (%)
Hadley et al,[60] 2012	7	Transanosphincteric	BT+EBRT (7)	Gracilis flap (1)	57
Mundy et al,[56] 2011	17	Abdominal SP (8) Perineal (3) Abdominoperineal (6)	BT (3) EBRT (4) BT+EBRT (10)	Omentum (15) Gracilis (2)	0
Lane et al,[32] 2006	13	Transanal (2) Perineal (11)	BT (5) EBRT (2) BT+EBRT (6)	Omentum (2) Gracilis flap (7)	100 Transanal, 0 Perineal
Vanni et al,[59] 2010	39	Perineal	BT (13) EBRT (7) BT+EBRT (12) BT+EBRT+CT (1) EBRT+HIFU (1) EBRT+CT (1) BT+HIFU (1) MT (1)	Gracilis flap (37) Gluteal flap (1) Singapore flap (1)	16
Elliot et al,[66] 2006	6	Transanal (1) Abdominal (1) Perineal (4)	EBRT+ CT (1) EBRT+TA (1) BT+EBRT (3) BT (1)	Dartos flap (1)	16

Abbreviations: CT, cryotherapy; MT, microwave therapy.

patients reported the incontinence as having a significant impact on QOL.

A similar study evaluated QOL in 25 patients following successful transperineal repair with gracilis muscle flap interposition for complex RUF.[78] RUF cause was radical prostatectomy in 8 (32%), radical prostatectomy plus EBRT in 8 (32%), EBRT plus BT in 4 (16%), EBRT alone in 3 (12%), and cryotherapy in 2 (8%). The patients completed a questionnaire concerning QOL, addressing urine and bowel function. Postoperative urinary continence was reported in 13 (52%) patients. An additional 5 (20%) patients required an AUS for a total of 18 (72%) reporting urinary continence. Regarding bowel function, 2 (8%) reported fecal incontinence, with 1 patient requiring neuromodulation and an artificial bowel sphincter. Three patients (12%) underwent permanent bladder and bowel diversion with an Indiana pouch and permanent colostomy. Although these two studies were of complex RUF of several different causes including radiation therapy for prostate cancer, the long-term success as gauged through QOL questionnaires of transperineal repair with gracilis muscle interposition was high. There are limited studies to conclude that RUF secondary to radiation therapy should be repaired with a specific approach. Nonetheless, the perineal approach

with gracilis interposition seems to have a high success of fistula closure as well as acceptable postoperative QOL concerning bowel and urinary function.

SUMMARY

Radiation-induced injury of the urinary tract is a complex issue that can lead to debilitating morbidity for the patient. Because of the small number of studies available addressing urethral stricture, BNC, and RUF, a consensus on the management and treatment algorithm has yet to be determined. Nonetheless, available studies indicate that successful reconstruction of these complex lower urinary tract injuries after radiation therapy can be performed.

REFERENCES

1. Dutreix J, Tubiana M, Pierquin B. The hazy dawn of brachytherapy. Radiother Oncol 1998;49(3): 223–32.
2. Young HH. The use of radium and the punch operation in desperate cases of enlarged prostate. Ann Surg 1917;65(5):633–41.
3. Aronowitz JN. Benjamin Barringer: originator of the transperineal prostate implant. Urology 2002;60(4): 731–4.

4. Nguyen PL, Zietman AL. High-dose external beam radiation for localized prostate cancer: current status and future challenges. Cancer J 2007;13(5): 295–301.

5. Mohler JL, Armstrong AJ, Bhanson RR, et al. Prostate cancer, version 3.2012: featured updates to the NCCN guidelines. J Natl Compr Canc Netw 2012;10(9):1081–7.

6. Thompson I, Thrasher JB, Aus G, et al. Guideline for the management of clinically localized prostate cancer: 2007 update. J Urol 2007;177(6):2106–31.

7. Cooperberg MR, Broering JM, Litwin MS, et al. The contemporary management of prostate cancer in the United States: lessons from the cancer of the prostate strategic urologic research endeavor (CapSURE), a national disease registry. J Urol 2004;171(4):1393–401.

8. Sheets NC, Goldin GH, Meyer AM, et al. Intensity-modulated radiation therapy, proton therapy, or conformal radiation therapy and morbidity and disease control in localized prostate cancer. JAMA 2012;307(15):1611–20.

9. Bolus NE. Basic review of radiation biology and terminology. J Nucl Med Technol 2001;29(2):67–73 [test: 76–7].

10. Tibbs MK. Wound healing following radiation therapy: a review. Radiother Oncol 1997;42(2):99–106.

11. Bernstein EF, Sullivan FJ, Mitchell JB, et al. Biology of chronic radiation effect on tissues and wound healing. Clin Plast Surg 1993;20(3):435–53.

12. Mundy AR, Andrich DE. Urethral strictures. BJU Int 2011;107(1):6–26.

13. Pieters BR, de Back DZ, Koning CC, et al. Comparison of three radiotherapy modalities on biochemical control and overall survival for the treatment of prostate cancer: a systematic review. Radiother Oncol 2009;93(2):168–73.

14. Khor R, Duchesne G, Tai KH, et al. Direct 2-arm comparison shows benefit of high-dose-rate brachytherapy boost vs external beam radiation therapy alone for prostate cancer. Int J Radiat Oncol Biol Phys 2013;85(3):679–85.

15. Viani GA, Pellizzon AC, Guimarães FS, et al. High dose rate and external beam radiotherapy in locally advanced prostate cancer. Am J Clin Oncol 2009;32(2):187–90.

16. Challapalli A, Jones E, Harvey C, et al. High dose rate prostate brachytherapy: an overview of the rationale, experience and emerging applications in the treatment of prostate cancer. Br J Radiol 2012;85(Spec No 1):S18–27.

17. Elliott SP, Meng MV, Elkin EP, et al. Incidence of urethral stricture after primary treatment for prostate cancer: data from CaPSURE. J Urol 2007;178(2):529–34 [discussion: 534].

18. Mohammed N, Kestin L, Ghilezan M, et al. Comparison of acute and late toxicities for three modern

high-dose radiation treatment techniques for localized prostate cancer. Int J Radiat Oncol Biol Phys 2012;82(1):204–12.

19. Sullivan L, Williams SG, Tai KH, et al. Urethral stricture following high dose rate brachytherapy for prostate cancer. Radiother Oncol 2009;91(2): 232–6.

20. Merrick GS, Butler WM, Tollenaar BG, et al. The dosimetry of prostate brachytherapy-induced urethral strictures. Int J Radiat Oncol Biol Phys 2002; 52(2):461–8.

21. Earley JJ, Abdelbaky AM, Cunningham MJ, et al. Correlation between prostate brachytherapy-related urethral stricture and peri-apical urethral dosimetry: a matched case-control study. Radiother Oncol 2012;104(2):187–91.

22. Hindson BR, Millar JL, Matheson B. Urethral strictures following high-dose-rate brachytherapy for prostate cancer: analysis of risk factors. Brachytherapy 2013;12(1):50–5.

23. Zelefsky MJ, Chan H, Hunt M, et al. Long-term outcome of high dose intensity modulated radiation therapy for patients with clinically localized prostate cancer. J Urol 2006;176(4 Pt 1):1415–9.

24. Sandhu AS, Zelefsky MJ, Lee HJ, et al. Long-term urinary toxicity after 3-dimensional conformal radiotherapy for prostate cancer in patients with prior history of transurethral resection. Int J Radiat Oncol Biol Phys 2000;48(3):643–7.

25. Ishiyama H, Hirayama T, Jhaveri P, et al. Is there an increase in genitourinary toxicity in patients treated with transurethral resection of the prostate and radiotherapy?: a systematic review. Am J Clin Oncol 2012. [Epub ahead of print].

26. Thompson IM Jr, Tangen CM, Paradelo J, et al. Adjuvant radiotherapy for pathologically advanced prostate cancer: a randomized clinical trial. JAMA 2006;296(19):2329–35.

27. Slater JD, Rossi CJ Jr, Yonemoto LT, et al. Proton therapy for prostate cancer: the initial Loma Linda University experience. Int J Radiat Oncol Biol Phys 2004;59(2):348–52.

28. Shipley WU, Verhey LJ, Munzenrider JE, et al. Advanced prostate cancer: the results of a randomized comparative trial of high dose irradiation boosting with conformal protons compared with conventional dose irradiation using photons alone. Int J Radiat Oncol Biol Phys 1995;32(1):3–12.

29. Sarosdy MF. Urinary and rectal complications of contemporary permanent transperineal brachytherapy for prostate carcinoma with or without external beam radiation therapy. Cancer 2004; 101(4):754–60.

30. Wallner K, Roy J, Harrison L. Tumor control and morbidity following transperineal iodine 125 implantation for stage T1/T2 prostatic carcinoma. J Clin Oncol 1996;14(2):449–53.

31. Zelefsky MJ, Wallner KE, Ling CC, et al. Comparison of the 5-year outcome and morbidity of three-dimensional conformal radiotherapy versus transperineal permanent iodine-125 implantation for early-stage prostatic cancer. J Clin Oncol 1999;17(2):517–22.

32. Lane BR, Stein DE, Remzi FH, et al. Management of radiotherapy induced rectourethral fistula. J Urol 2006;175(4):1382–7 [discussion: 1387-8].

33. Pisansky TM, Kozelsky TF, Myers RP, et al. Radiotherapy for isolated serum prostate specific antigen elevation after prostatectomy for prostate cancer. J Urol 2000;163(3):845–50.

34. Huang EH, Pollack A, Levy L, et al. Late rectal toxicity: dose-volume effects of conformal radiotherapy for prostate cancer. Int J Radiat Oncol Biol Phys 2002;54(5):1314–21.

35. Hu K, Wallner K. Clinical course of rectal bleeding following I-125 prostate brachytherapy. Int J Radiat Oncol Biol Phys 1998;41(2):263–5.

36. Theodorescu D, Gillenwater JY, Koutrouvelis PG. Prostatourethral-rectal fistula after prostate brachytherapy. Cancer 2000;89(10):2085–91.

37. Stone NN, Stock RG. Complications following permanent prostate brachytherapy. Eur Urol 2002; 41(4):427–33.

38. Chrouser KL, Leibovich BC, Sweat SD, et al. Urinary fistulas following external radiation or permanent brachytherapy for the treatment of prostate cancer. J Urol 2005;173(6):1953–7.

39. Vallancien G, Gupta R, Cathelineau X, et al. Initial results of salvage laparoscopic radical prostatectomy after radiation failure. J Urol 2003;170(5):1838–40.

40. Gotto GT, Yunis LH, Vora K, et al. Impact of prior prostate radiation on complications after radical prostatectomy. J Urol 2010;184(1):136–42.

41. Nguyen PL, D'Amico AV, Lee AK, et al. Patient selection, cancer control, and complications after salvage local therapy for postradiation prostate-specific antigen failure: a systematic review of the literature. Cancer 2007;110(7):1417–28.

42. Miller RJ Jr, Cohen JK, Shuman B, et al. Percutaneous, transperineal cryosurgery of the prostate as salvage therapy for post radiation recurrence of adenocarcinoma. Cancer 1996;77(8):1510–4.

43. Pisters LL, von Eschenbach AC, Scott SM, et al. The efficacy and complications of salvage cryotherapy of the prostate. J Urol 1997;157(3):921–5.

44. Ghafar MA, Johnson CW, De La Taille A, et al. Salvage cryotherapy using an argon based system for locally recurrent prostate cancer after radiation therapy: the Columbia experience. J Urol 2001; 166(4):1333–7 [discussion: 1337-8].

45. Bahn DK, Lee F, Silverman P, et al. Salvage cryosurgery for recurrent prostate cancer after radiation therapy: a seven-year follow-up. Clin Prostate Cancer 2003;2(2):111–4.

46. Han KR, Cohen JK, Miller RJ, et al. Treatment of organ confined prostate cancer with third generation cry surgery: preliminary multicenter experience. J Ur 2003;170(4 Pt 1):1126–30.

47. Wong WW, Buskirk SJ, Schild SE, et al. Combine prostate brachytherapy and short-term androge deprivation therapy as salvage therapy for loca recurrent prostate cancer after external beam irr diation. J Urol 2006;176(5):2020–4.

48. Lee B, Shinohara K, Weinberg V, et al. Feasibility high-dose-rate brachytherapy salvage for loc prostate cancer recurrence after radiotherapy: th University of California-San Francisco experienc Int J Radiat Oncol Biol Phys 2007;67(4):1106–12

49. Nguyen PL, Chen MH, D'Amico AV, et al. Magnet resonance image-guided salvage brachytherap after radiation in select men who initially presente with favorable-risk prostate cancer: a prospecti phase 2 study. Cancer 2007;110(7):1485–92.

50. Jackson MJ, Sciberras J, Mangera A, et a Defining a patient-reported outcome measure f urethral stricture surgery. Eur Urol 2011;60(1):60–

51. Heyns CF, Marais DC. Prospective evaluation of th American Urological Association symptom inde and peak urinary flow rate for the followup of me with known urethral stricture disease. J Urol 200 168(5):2051–4.

52. Westney OL. Salvage surgery for bladder outl obstruction after prostatectomy or cystectom Curr Opin Urol 2008;18(6):570–4.

53. Mundy AR, Andrich DE. Posterior urethral comp cations of the treatment of prostate cancer. BJ Int 2012;110(3):304–25.

54. Rule AD, Jacobson DJ, McGree ME, et al. Longit dinal changes in post-void residual and voided vc ume among community dwelling men. J Urol 200 174(4 Pt 1):1317–21 [discussion: 1321-2; auth reply: 1322].

55. McAninch JW, Laing FC, Jeffrey RB Jr. Sonouret rography in the evaluation of urethral strictures: preliminary report. J Urol 1988;139(2):294–7.

56. Mundy AR, Andrich DE. Urorectal fistulae followir the treatment of prostate cancer. BJU Int 201 107(8):1298–303.

57. Turina M, Mulhall AM, Mahid SS, et al. Frequenc and surgical management of chronic complicatior related to pelvic radiation. Arch Surg 2008;143(1 46–52 [discussion: 52].

58. Larson DW, Chrouser K, Young-Fadok T, et a Rectal complications after modern radiation f prostate cancer: a colorectal surgical challeng J Gastrointest Surg 2005;9(4):461–6.

59. Vanni AJ, Buckley JC, Zinman LN. Management surgical and radiation induced rectourethral fi tulas with an interposition muscle flap and selecti buccal mucosal onlay graft. J Urol 2010;184(6 2400–4.

60. Hadley DA, Southwick A, Middleton RG. York-Mason procedure for repair of recto-urinary fistulae: a 40-year experience. BJU Int 2012;109(7):1095–8.

61. Zinman L. The management of the complex recto-urethral fistula. BJU Int 2004;94(9):1212–3.

62. Meeks JJ, Brandes SB, Morey AF, et al. Urethroplasty for radiotherapy induced bulbomembranous strictures: a multi-institutional experience. J Urol 2011;185(5):1761–5.

63. Erickson BA, Granieri MA, Meeks JJ, et al. Prospective analysis of erectile dysfunction after anterior urethroplasty: incidence and recovery of function. J Urol 2010;183(2):657–61.

64. Erickson BA, Granieri MA, Meeks JJ, et al. Prospective analysis of ejaculatory function after anterior urethral reconstruction. J Urol 2010;184(1): 238–42.

65. Merrick GS, Butler WM, Wallner KE, et al. Risk factors for the development of prostate brachytherapy related urethral strictures. J Urol 2006;175(4): 1376–80 [discussion: 1381].

66. Elliott SP, McAninch JW, Chi T, et al. Management of severe urethral complications of prostate cancer therapy. J Urol 2006;176(6 Pt 1):2508–13.

67. Glass AS, McAninch JW, Zaid UB, et al. Urethroplasty after radiation therapy for prostate cancer. Urology 2012;79(6):1402–5.

68. Mundy AR. Anastomotic urethroplasty. BJU Int 2005;96(6):921–44.

69. Kaffenberger SD, Keegan KA, Bansal NK, et al. Salvage robotic-assisted laparoscopic radical prostatectomy: a single institution, five-year experience. J Urol 2013;189(2):507–13.

70. Schlossberg S, Jordan G, Schellhammer P. Repair of obliterative vesicourethral stricture after radical prostatectomy: a technique for preservation of continence. Urology 1995;45(3):510–3.

71. Wessells H, Morey AF, McAninch JW. Obliterative vesicourethral strictures following radical prostatectomy for prostate cancer: reconstructive armamentarium. J Urol 1998;160(4):1373–5.

72. Pfalzgraf D, Beuke M, Isbarn H, et al. Open retropubic reanastomosis for highly recurrent and complex bladder neck stenosis. J Urol 2011;186(5): 1944–7.

73. Simonato A, Ennas M, Benelli A, et al. Comparison between two different two-stage transperineal approaches to treat urethral strictures or bladder neck contracture associated with severe urinary incontinence that occurred after pelvic surgery: report of our experience. Adv Urol 2012;2012: 481943.

74. Thomas C, Jones J, Jäger W, et al. Incidence, clinical symptoms and management of rectourethral fistulas after radical prostatectomy. J Urol 2010; 183(2):608–12.

75. Rivera R, Barboglio PG, Hellinger M, et al. Staging rectourinary fistulas to guide surgical treatment. J Urol 2007;177(2):586–8.

76. Dal Moro F, Secco S, Valotto C, et al. Twenty-year experience with surgical management of rectourinary fistulas by posterior sagittal transrectal approach (York-Mason). Surgery 2011;150(5): 975–9.

77. Garofalo TE, Delaney CP, Jones SM, et al. Rectal advancement flap repair of rectourethral fistula: a 20-year experience. Dis Colon Rectum 2003; 46(6):762–9.

78. Ghoniem G, Elmissiry M, Weiss E, et al. Transperineal repair of complex rectourethral fistula using gracilis muscle flap interposition–can urinary and bowel functions be preserved? J Urol 2008; 179(5):1882–6.

79. Samplaski MK, Wood HM, Lane BR, et al. Functional and quality-of-life outcomes in patients undergoing transperineal repair with gracilis muscle interposition for complex rectourethral fistula. Urology 2011;77(3):736–41.

Penile Prosthesis Insertion for Acute Priapism

Timothy J. Tausch, MD[a],*, Ryan Mauck, MD[b],
Lee C. Zhao, MD[b], Allen F. Morey, MD[b]

KEYWORDS

- Priapism • Penile prosthesis • Priapistic episode

KEY POINTS

- Shunt surgery is not universally successful toward detumescence, may lead to erectile dysfunction, and can make eventual penile prosthesis insertion difficult.
- Penile prosthesis insertion during a priapistic episode alleviates ischemic pain, allows the patient to resume sexual function sooner, and prevents corporal scarring and shortening that makes subsequent prosthesis implantation difficult.

INTRODUCTION

Priapism is defined as a full or partial erection that continues more than 4 hours beyond sexual stimulation and orgasm or is unrelated to sexual stimulation. Two broad, cause-derived categories guide management strategies. Ischemic (or veno-occlusive, low-flow) priapism warrants immediate intervention, whereas nonischemic (arterial, high-flow) priapism does not.

The erection in ischemic priapism is marked by profound, unremitting venous congestion that creates a compartment syndrome that ultimately prevents arterial inflow. Corporal blood gas studies have shown that ischemia and acidosis can occur within 6 hours of a priapism episode.[1] Although erectile dysfunction rates approach 25% to 50% in patients with ischemic priapism, those with an episode greater than 24 hours typically face invasive shunt procedures, prolonged pain, and a 90% risk of subsequent erectile dysfunction.[2–4]

The delayed sequelae of prolonged ischemia and acidosis frequently result in corporal fibrosis and penile shortening. Therefore, placement of the prosthesis in the acute setting is easier than delayed implantation.[3] In patients with prolonged episodes of acute priapism, early implantation alleviates ischemic pain, allows the patient to resume sexual function sooner, and prevents the corporal scarring and shortening that makes subsequent prosthesis implantation difficult.

PATIENT EVALUATION OVERVIEW

When the persistent erection is accompanied by pain, ischemia should be suspected, because nonischemic priapism is generally not painful. A careful history may reveal predisposing factors, such as sickle cell hemoglobinopathy (or other hematologic conditions), neurologic disease, or pharmacologic reasons for the erection. Pelvic and perineal trauma can result in nonischemic priapism.

On physical examination, inspection and palpation reveal rigid corpora cavernosa, with soft corpus spongiosum and glans tissues. Laboratory testing can detect hematologic abnormalities, and in African American men without a known history of sickle cell disease, a sickle cell preparation and hemoglobin electrophoresis should be obtained. Corporal blood gas analysis can differentiate ischemic from nonischemic priapism, with ischemic blood revealing acidosis, hypercarbia, and hypoxia.

a Madigan Army Medical Center, 9040A Jackson Avenue, Tacoma, WA 98431, USA; b Department of Urology, UT Southwestern, 5323 Harry Hines Boulevard, Dallas, TX 75390, USA
* Corresponding author.
E-mail address: tjtausch@gmail.com

Urol Clin N Am 40 (2013) 421–425
http://dx.doi.org/10.1016/j.ucl.2013.04.010
0094-0143/13/$ – see front matter Published by Elsevier Inc.

PHARMACOLOGIC TREATMENT OPTIONS

Initial therapy involves corporal aspiration, irrigation, and injection of α-adrenergic agonists, with the intent of relaxing the smooth muscle and re-establishing arterial inflow, venous drainage, and subsequent detumescence. This approach is highly effective, especially in cases of less than 24 hours' duration.[5,6]

When priapism is not effectively treated in a prompt manner, irreversible fibrosis develops. Thus, up to 25% of patients with priapism experience chronic erectile dysfunction.[7] Irreversible fibrotic changes occurring after 48 hours stem from smooth muscle cell necrosis within the corpora cavernosa and subsequent transformation into fibroblastlike cells.[8,9] The corporal scarring is irreversible and leads to permanent erectile dysfunction that is refractory to medical management and renders delayed surgical placement of a penile prosthesis technically challenging.

SURGICAL TREATMENT OPTIONS

For priapism that is refractory to medical management, corpora-spongiosal shunts are usually performed.[10,11] There is no general consensus on the management of refractory or delayed cases of ischemic priapism. Immediate insertion of a penile prosthesis is an emerging, effective therapeutic concept in the urological armamentarium.

HISTORICAL PERSPECTIVE ON PROSTHETIC IMPLANTATION

Most initial reports and series for prosthetic insertion for priapism have involved patients with sickle cell trait, delayed and/or recurrent presentation, or failure of previous shunt surgeries. Early reports describe the use of semirigid devices, which were theoretically superior to inflatable devices due to the need to overcome significant corporal rigidity.[12,13] Surgeons encounter technical challenges with the procedure because of the fibrosis, necessitating corporal tunneling and excavation, with high risk for further interventions.[14]

EARLY IMPLANTATION

In 1996, Monga and colleagues[15] introduced the concept of managing potency and recurrence in sickle cell patients with "early" implantation. Rees and colleagues[1] effectively managed 8 patients with ischemic priapism of a mean duration of 91 hours with the insertion of either malleable or inflatable devices. Four (50%) of the patients had failed previous shunts. Only one failure was reported, with penile deformity caused by

compression of an inflatable cylinder by fibrosi leading the authors to conclude that a semirig device was best used as a temporizing measur thereby preserving penile length and corpor patency until an inflatable device can be offered

COMPLICATIONS

Immediate implantation of a penile prosthesis not without its risks. In one series, infectior occurred in 6%.[16] In the same series, 12% unde went elective exchange for inflatable penile pro thesis; other revision procedures were needed 12%, and 6% had impending distal erosion of th malleable device requiring replacement with a inflatable device. An important factor in outcome is the use of surgical interventions before devic implantation. It is accepted that ischemic priapisr that does not respond to medical therapy shou be treated with a shunt, and the 2003 America Urological Association Guidelines recommen reserving shunt procedures until after an adequa attempt to treat with sympathomimetic injec tions.[17] By compromising corporal integrity, suc interventions may expose patients to increase risk of complications, from the shunt procedure i self or if immediate prosthetic insertion is offerec

Apical shunts for ischemic priapism would seer to increase the risk of apical perforation durin corporal dilation and subsequent prosthesis extru sion. However, in a series of 12 patients wh presented with prolonged ischemic priapism, 1 of whom had undergone unsuccessful shunt su gery, Salem and Aasser reported successful im mediate insertion of malleable prostheses in a patients, with only one unilateral corporal perfora tion that was managed intraoperatively.[2] The avoided distal protrusion by fixing the cylinder to the edges of the tunicae albuginea with nonat sorbable sling sutures at the site of the corporo omy. With a mean follow-up of 15 months, a patients were satisfied and there were no dista erosions noted. Sedigh and colleagues[3] reporte 5 patients who had failed distal shunt surger and underwent immediate insertion of inflatabl devices, and all patients had acceptable out comes. All 5 experienced a decrease in penil sensitivity that resolved at 3 months, and all wer satisfied with the results of surgery based on Inter national Index of Erectile Function Questionnaire answers (mean value of 4).

TIMING OF SURGERY

There is no consensus on appropriate timing c penile prosthesis insertion, and one must weig this factor carefully given the irreversible natur f the therapy. Most authors agree that irreversible corporal damage occurs within 24 to 48 hours of ischemic priapism, with eventual, unavoidable erectile dysfunction. Immediate insertion of a penile prosthesis should be discussed with these patients, given the benefits to sexual function, penile length, and surgical technique. Some authors suggest a delay of 1 week to appropriately counsel patients and allow for better understanding, but the delay should not exceed 20 days, as the patients who delayed experienced an average penile shortening of 3.5 cm due to severe fibrosis, and the implantations were significantly more difficult.[3]

Moreover, one may question the need for shunt altogether in select cases. Shunt surgery, although an integral component of the treatment algorithm, has a high failure rate with long-term consequences. Nixon and colleagues[18] found that nearly 50% of patients undergoing initial shunt surgery required additional procedures to achieve detumescence, with 90% reporting significant erectile dysfunction. In patients with prior episodes of erectile dysfunction or medical comorbidity, such as sickle cell disease, failure of aspiration and irrigation may warrant prosthetic placement, given the recurrent nature of the disease process.[19] Conversely, the authors have observed that the long corporotomies performed during acute insertion of prosthetic cylinders function impressively

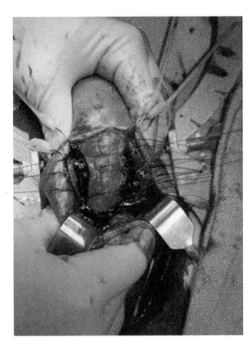

Fig. 2. Removal of old clot.

as an immediate surgical shunt, leading promptly to healthy arterial inflow.

SURGICAL TECHNIQUE

A 2-in longitudinal penoscrotal incision is made—this is longer than the incision normally used for penile implant insertion because a longer corporotomy is required to insert the prosthesis. Patients with ischemic priapism often have significant edema of the penile skin, from both the disease process and the efforts of corporal irrigation. An incision in the scrotum instead of on the penis avoids the edematous penile skin and is a less apparent scar. Blunt dissection is performed

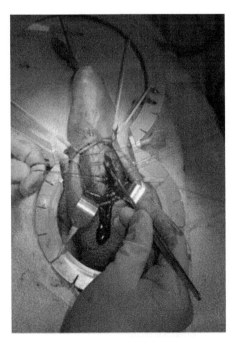

Fig. 1. Incision of corporal cavernosa with outflow of ischemic blood.

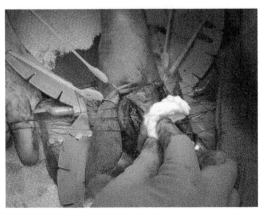

Fig. 3. Arterial blood return.

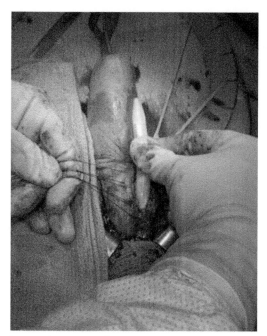

Fig. 4. Placement of malleable penile prosthesis—note that the device is deliberately undersized by 1 cm, extending only to the coronal sulcus.

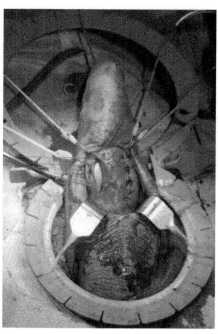

Fig. 5. Corporotomy closure.

to reveal the corporal bodies. A self-retaining ring retractor system is used for exposure. Traction sutures with 2-0 polydioxanone are placed on the corporal bodies—the authors use 3 paired traction sutures on each corpora. An incision is made on the corpora (Fig. 1), with return of clotted blood.

Manual compression of the penis may be performed to remove the clot (Fig. 2). Corporal dilation is performed, being especially careful if a shunt had been performed distally. Dilation results in the return of bright red, arterial, blood flow (Fig. 3). The corporotomies and wound are irrigated with antibiotic irrigation. A semirigid penile prosthesis is placed (Fig. 4)—it is essential not to

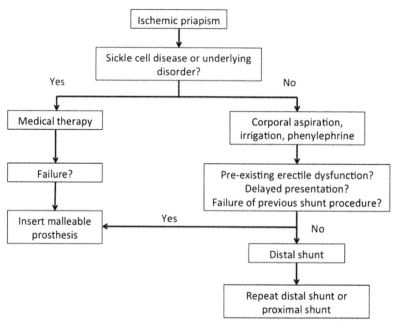

Management algorithm for acute ischemic priapism.

ze the cylinder length aggressively as one would ormally do for inflatable device insertion; the uthors measure the corporal length only to the oronal sulcus, deliberately undersizing by 1 cm. action sutures are then tied together to close e corporotomy (**Fig. 5**). The authors often prefer 9-mm cylinder diameter in many cases because the potential difficulty closing the corporotomy ue to surrounding congestion and fibrosis. The cision is closed in multiple layers with absorb-ole suture. It is the authors' practice not to leave ains.

UMMARY

reasonable option for treatment of prolonged or fractory ischemic priapism is early implantation a penile prosthesis, with the advantages of pres-vation of sexual function, prevention of penile hortening, and relative procedural ease. Timing the procedure is controversial and warrants areful patient counseling regarding the risks, ben-its, level of motivation for subsequent sexual ac-vity, and expectations of any treatment decision.

EFERENCES

1. Rees RW, Kalsi J, Minhas S, et al. The management of low-flow priapism with the immediate insertion of a penile prosthesis. BJU Int 2002;90:893–7.

2. Salem EA, El Aasser O. Management of ischemic priapism by penile prosthesis insertion: prevention of distal erosion. J Urol 2010;183:2300–3.

3. Sedigh O, Rolle L, Negro CL, et al. Early insertion of inflatable prosthesis for intractable ischemic pria-pism: our experience and review of the literature. Int J Impot Res 2011;23:158–64.

4. El-Bahnasawy MS, Dawood A, Farouk A. Low-flow priapism: risk factors for erectile dysfunction. BJU Int 2002;89:285–90.

5. Pohl J, Pott B, Kleinhans G. Priapism: a three-phase concept of management according to aetiology and prognosis. Br J Urol 1986;58:113–8.

6. Broderick GA, Harkaway R. Pharmacologic erection: time-dependent changes in the corporal environ-ment. Int J Impot Res 1994;6:9–16.

7. Nehra A. Priapism. Pathophysiology and non-surgical management. In: Porst H, Buvat J, editors. Standard practice in sexual medicine. Boston: Blackwell Publishing; 2006. p. 174–9.

8. Spycher MA, Hauri D. The ultrastructure of the erec-tile tissue in priapism. J Urol 1986;135:142–7.

9. Ul-Hasan M, El-Sakka AI, Lee C, et al. Expression of TGF-beta-1 mRNA and ultrastructural alterations in pharmacologically induced prolonged penile erec-tion in a canine model. J Urol 1998;160:2263–6.

10. Lue TF, Pescatori ES. Distal cavernosum-glans shunts for ischemic priapism. J Sex Med 2006;3: 749–52.

11. Burnett AL. Surgical management of ischemic pria-pism. J Sex Med 2012;9:114–20.

12. Kelami A. Implantation of Small-Carrion prosthesis in the treatment of erectile impotence after priapism: difficulties and effects. Urol Int 1985;40:343–6.

13. Bertram RA, Carson CC 3rd, Webster GD. Implanta-tion of penile prostheses in patients impotent after priapism. Urology 1985;26:325–7.

14. Douglas L, Fletcher H, Serjeant GR. Penile prostheses in the management of impotence in sickle cell disease. Br J Urol 1990;65:533–5.

15. Monga M, Broderick GA, Hellstrom WJ. Priapism in sickle cell disease: the case for early implantation of the penile prosthesis. Eur Urol 1996;30:54–9.

16. Ralph DJ, Garaffa G, Muneer A, et al. The immediate insertion of a penile prosthesis for acute ischaemic priapism. Eur Urol 2009;56:1033–8.

17. Montague DK, Jarow J, Broderick GA, et al. American Urological Association guideline on the management of priapism. J Urol 2003;170:1318–24.

18. Nixon RG, O'Connor JL, Milam DF. Efficacy of shunt surgery for refractory low flow priapism: a report on the incidence of failed detumescence and erectile dysfunction. J Urol 2003;170:883–6.

19. Tausch TJ, Evans LA, Morey AF. Immediate insertion of a semirigid penile prosthesis for refractory ischemic priapism. Mil Med 2007;172:1211–2.

Advances in Diagnosis and Management of Genital Injuries

Andrew J. Chang, MD*, Steven B. Brandes, MD

KEYWORDS

• Genital • Penile • Scrotal • Testicular • Injuries • Trauma • Amputation • Burn

KEY POINTS

- External genital trauma is uncommon and rarely life-threatening but warrants prompt evaluation for proper management.
- The treating physician should have a high index of suspicion when evaluating genital trauma.
- A missed diagnosis can lead to undue, long-term morbidity.
- The treating physician should be selective in obtaining imaging studies based on mechanism of injury and presenting symptoms.
- The primary goal of reconstructive surgery is to preserve tissue, cosmesis, and function.

INTRODUCTION

External genital trauma is uncommon but can cause devastating long-term physical, psychological, and functional quality-of-life consequences. Therefore, the treating physician must be able to diagnose the injury in a timely fashion and be knowledgeable of principles of delayed reconstruction. In the civilian population, genital trauma is roughly 45% penetrating, 45% blunt, and 10% burns and industrial accidents.[1] The most important objective of management is preserving genital function and cosmesis, while minimizing long-term sequelae.

GENITAL AND PERINEAL BURNS

Burns of the genitalia and perineum require referral to a burn center, are rarely isolated, and typically involve other areas of the body. The genitalia alone only comprise 1% of total body surface area (TBSA), and studies have demonstrated an average TBSA of 21% to 56% for all patients with perineal burns.[2–4] Initial management of perineal burns is removal of all clothing, rapid and aggressive fluid and electrolyte replacement, and Foley or suprapubic tube placement to monitor sufficient urine output. Evaluation includes a complete physical examination, laboratory evaluation with urinalysis, tetanus prophylaxis, intravenous antibiotics, and an estimate of extent and depth of the burn (TBSA) involved. Burns should be treated according to the mechanism of injury and depth of injury.[1] Genital burns demand very close observation and admission to an intensive care unit or burn unit.

BURN CLASSIFICATION/DEPTH OF BURN

First-degree burns affect the epidermis only and are characterized by pink color, with minimal histologic damage, but significant pain. First-degree burns usually do not have long-term scarring. Second-degree burns are divided into superficial partial thickness and deep partial thickness. Superficial partial-thickness burns involve the epidermis and the papillary dermis and present as pink, moist, tender skin with thin-walled blisters. Deep partial-thickness burns include the reticular

Disclosures: None.
Division of Urologic Surgery, Washington University School of Medicine, 4960 Children's Place, Campus Box 8242, St Louis, MO 63110, USA
* Corresponding author.
E-mail address: changa@wudosis.wustl.edu

urologic.theclinics.com

dermis and present with mottled red and blanched white skin with thick-walled blisters and tender skin. Third-degree burns are full-thickness burns that destroy the epidermis and the entirety of the dermis. Third-degree burns are characterized by a waxy-white or black, dry skin that is insensate.[5]

THERMAL BURNS

Thermal burns of the genitals are caused mainly by flame, but also by boiling water or grease (with scald). Genital burns are typically first-degree and second-degree burns that can be treated without debridement and require only a topical antimicrobial ointment, usually 1% silver sulfadiazine. Genital third-degree burns should be treated with prompt surgical intervention, as conservative management only leads to increased incidence of infection, longer recovery time and hospital stays, and burn scar contracture.

Third-degree burns to the scrotum should be promptly débrided of all nonviable tissue and then immediately skin grafted. With immediate treatment, infection is usually not an issue and there is no reason for delay in scrotal reconstruction with thigh pouch creation.

The penile skin is very thin and thus vulnerable to full-thickness, third-degree burns. Should this occur, the nonviable skin should be sharply débrided; the wound should be primarily closed, and skin should be grafted to the denuded site (**Fig. 1**). For circumferential penile injury, severe lymphatic obstruction and lymphedema can occur, so all skin distal from the injury site to the subcorona should be excised. Owing to the tremendous vascularity, burns to the glans usually do not need debridement unless it is clearly necrotic.[6] Patients with third-degree burns to the glans or the ventral shaft of the penis should have suprapubic tubes rather than Foley catheters. Foley catheters can cause pressure necrosis resulting in severe hypospadias due to anterior urethral slough, especially when left in a dependent position.

Thermal burns have the potential for long-term sequelae by urethral slough, urethral stenosis, and eventually scar contracture at 3 to 6 months postinjury. These wounds are managed with surgical release and skin grafts.

CHEMICAL BURNS

Chemical burns should be managed with immediate removal of any clothing and aggressive flushing with copious amounts of sterile water. However, do not peel off adherent clothing. Duration of exposure and concentration of the chemical are directly proportional to the extent of the injury. Searching for neutralizing agent is not necessary, as time is of the essence for these patients; most are best served with sterile water irrigation.

ELECTRICAL BURNS

Electrical burns can be devastating, as the degree and the depth of the burn can be deceiving. The damage is often beyond what is obviously visible on the surface and an extensive exploration of the deep and surrounding structures are warranted to evaluate the extent of the injury. A thorough workup for electrical burns include examination for any related bladder, rectum, pelvic organ, or skeletal damage by cystoscopy, sigmoidoscopy, vaginal speculum examination (if applicable), and pelvic radiograph. Urinalysis must be obtained for hemoglobinuria and myoglobinuria, as their presence can cause acute renal damage. When present, management should include aggressive hydration along with urine alkalization. Moreover, as cardiac arrhythmias and arrests have been known to be caused by electrical injuries, cardiac monitoring is also warranted. These burns can be managed in the same manner as a thermal burn, with prompt debridement, primary wound closure, and skin grafting. However, these burns are unique in needing additional debridement, often because of the extended damage. With serial debridements, these wounds can be eventually covered with skin grafts, without additional complications. At times, the debridement can be extensive, and bone or major vasculature is exposed in the wound. Myocutaneous flaps for coverage may be necessary at that point.

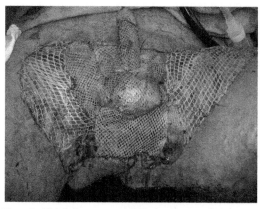

Fig. 1. Third-degree genital burn to the penis, scrotum, and inner thigh with meshed split-thickness grafts to cover the denuded area.

ANIMAL AND HUMAN BITES

Animal bites to the external genitalia are rare. Dog bites are the most common cause of injury and children are the most common victims. Initial management should include copious irrigation with saline and providone-iodine solution, debridement, broad spectrum antibiotic prophylaxis, tetnus-rabies immunizations (when appropriate), and immediate/early closure of wound. Infections after dog bites are rare, but treatment is sought soon after the event.[7] Recommended antibiotic therapies include β-lactam antibiotics with β-lactamase inhibitor (eg, amoxicillin-clavulanate), second-generation cephalosporins (eg, cefotetan, cefoxitin), or clindamycin with fluoroquinolones.[8]

Most human bite victims seek medical care after substantial delay and are more likely to present with gross infection of their wound than with a dog bite. Human bites are contaminated wounds that should never be closed primarily. Empiric antibiotic therapy of choice includes amoxicillin-clavulanate or moxifloxacin.[9]

SCROTAL DEGLOVING INJURIES

Due to the pendulous nature of the male genitalia and the laxity of the covering skin, the scrotum has tremendous capacity to resist injury. The skin, however, remains vulnerable to degloving injuries (**Fig. 2**). In the past, most degloving injuries were caused by agricultural ("power takeoff") and manufacturing machinery, but the incidence has decreased considerably with improved safety measures. Most present-day genital skin avulsion is due to motorcycle or bicycle accidents.

Avulsion injuries are usually along the fascial planes, often torn free without damage to the underlying tunica vaginalis or dartos fascia.[10] The scrotal skin is very compliant, redundant, and elastic and so defects with up to even 60% skin loss can be primarily closed.[11] To help prevent scrotal bleeding/hematoma after injury, a 2-layered closure of the deep fascia and skin is performed with an interlocking, running, absorbable suture. A scrotal drain after repair is controversial because resultant scrotal hematomas are usually in the interstitium of the skin and are not hematoceles.[12] However, if hemostasis is not possible or the patient has a coagulopathy, either a Penrose drain or a closed suction drain (eg, a Blake drain) is recommended. An antibacterial gauze dressing, such as xeroform, with fluff gauze and a compressive scrotal support should be placed to promote comfort and to facilitate healing.

If blunt traumatic scrotal skin loss is extensive (greater than 60%), several options are available for coverage. Repair should be performed without delay if the injury to the scrotum is not contaminated. Local skin flaps are all preferred options for coverage. When additional coverage is needed, split thickness skin grafting is the repair of choice, because it yields excellent cosmetic and functional outcome (**Fig. 3**).[13] Other ancillary measures include autologous skin grafts and tissue expanders. To begin the procedure, the testicles and cords are sutured together in the midline with multiple 3-0 polyglactin (Vicryl; Ethicon, Somerville, NJ, USA) sutures to create a singular structure, to ease skin grafting. The thick split-thickness skin graft is then harvested with a dermatome at 15 to 18

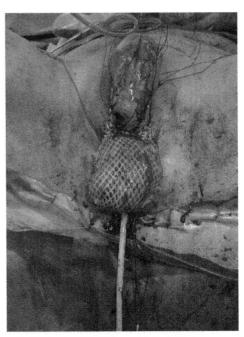

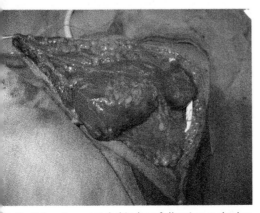

Fig. 2. Extensive scrotal skin loss following a degloving injury.

Fig. 3. Meshed split-thickness skin graft to cover the scrotum.

thousandths of an inch, ideally from the inner thigh, and meshed 1.5:1. Skin grafts to the penis are typically performed with nonmeshed grafts for both cosmesis and erectile function. For the scrotum, meshed grafts are used as the meshing simulates rugae, while allowing exudates to escape, thus improving graft take. The graft is then applied to cover the testes and cords and sutured in place at the perineum and ventral penile base. Multiple interrupted chromic sutures are placed in the graft to "quilt" it to the underlying tissue. The "neoscrotum" is then covered with xeroform, mineral oil–soaked cotton batting, and fluff gauze bandage. Bolster sutures of purple-dyed 2-0 Vicryl are then placed at the graft margins and tied over the dressings to facilitate immobilization. An easier-to-apply and quicker alternative to a bolster dressing is the use of a negative pressure wound therapy device (refer to section Management of Complex Urologic Wounds). Postoperatively, the patient is typically kept on bed rest for 48 hours (to prevent graft movement and allow for maximal imbibitions) and the dressings are removed on postoperative day 5. The patient then showers twice a day with soap and water, using a blow dryer on cool or gently patting the graft or harvest site with a towel to dry the graft.[12]

If the circumstances of the injury prevent immediate repair of the scrotum, the testicle should be wrapped in saline-soaked gauze for protection until surgery.[14] If definitive reconstruction is going to be delayed or the genital and perineal skin defects

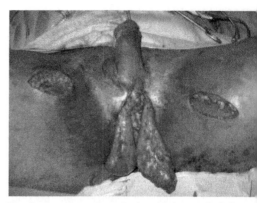

Fig. 5. Creation of testicular thigh pouch followin scrotal avulsion injury.

are very large, the testicles may be protected superficial thigh pouches as long as necessa (**Figs. 4** and **5**).[15] Thigh pouches not only prote the testes but augment future scrotal reconstruc tion, reduce the size of the perineal skin defe via secondary intention closure, and lighten th burden of labor-intensive and dressing change that are often very painful to the patient. Thig pouches prevent the testes and cord from formin a thick, fibrous, infected rind of granulation tissu Should this "rind" of granulation tissue form, must be completely removed down to the spe matic fascia and tunica for skin graft to take. Th rind is chronically infected tissue and is a po bed for skin graft to take. If the rind is left in sit the neoscrotum becomes contracted and fla tened out into an abnormal, nondependent pos tion. Care must be taken to avoid transmission the infection to the thigh region, so gross contam ination must be eliminated beforehand.

To create thigh pouches, the testis and cord ar initially dissected to the level of the external rin To prevent stretching of the spermatic cord wit thigh abduction, subcutaneous tissue pockets the fascia of the thighs should be dissected a far posteriorly and caudally as possible to allo for slack in the cord. Next, the fascia lata of th thigh is identified and then the pouch is dissecte superficial to the fascia lata with a sponge stic and 2 narrow deavers into the anterior thigh. the testes are placed too medially, it may caus pain and discomfort when patients adduct the legs. The plane usually dissects out easily an bluntly. Placing the testes and cord directly o top of the fascia lata facilitates mobilization for de layed scrotal reconstruction.

PENILE DEGLOVING INJURIES

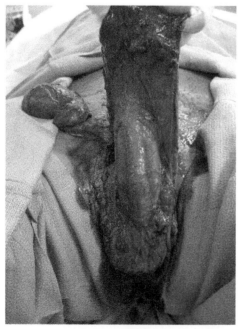

Fig. 4. Extensive penile and scrotal skin loss following a degloving injury.

Penile degloving injuries typically require immedi ate reconstruction and should be treated with ense of urgency owing to the nature of their function. Similar to the repair of the scrotum, primary closure of the skin should be attempted. Primary closure of the penis is often difficult, because the shaft skin is not as elastic or as redundant as scrotal skin. Not infrequently, the penile skin defect is circumferential, disrupting distal lymphatic drainage. With circumferential avulsion, the remaining skin distally must be excised to the subcorona to prevent chronic, disfiguring lymphedema.

The primary objective of reconstruction is to preserve erectile function. If a primary closure is not feasible, a thick nonmeshed split-thickness skin graft should be placed because it is less likely to contract (**Fig. 6**). Meshed split-thickness skin grafts on the penis can occasionally contract to the extent that erections become impaired. The skin graft should be wrapped around the penis with the seam on the ventral aspect of the shaft, to simulate a median raphé, while avoiding chordee. (Skin grafts placed on the penis shaft never regain normal sensation. However, sexual function is often preserved due the intact sensation in the glans.[16]) The graft is temporarily held in place with staples, and then quilting sutures (interrupted 3-0 chromic suture) are placed. At the proximal and distal aspect of the penis, 4 sutures of long, purple-dyed 2-0 Vicryl are placed circumferentially to tie over a bolster dressing.

The layers of dressing placed on top of the skin graft around the penis are Xeroform gauze, followed by a layer of mineral oil–soaked cotton wadding, fluff gauze, and then a compressive wrap of elastic bandage (conform). The long, purple-dyed stay sutures are then tied down to hold this bolster fixed in place (**Fig. 7**). Postoperatively, the patient is kept at bed rest for 48 hours, and the dressing removed at approximately postoperative day 5. These instructions are then followed by twice-daily showers and gentle drying of the graft with the cool setting of a hair dryer. An alternative, simpler way to immobilize the skin

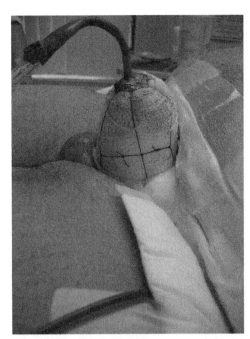

Fig. 7. "Penis-house" following skin grafting of penis.

graft is to wrap the fluff dressing with elastic bandage (conform) and staple the conform periodically while wrapping it around the penis, leaving the glans exposed. The final tight dressing is stapled at the edges of the skin.

If the patient is impotent and elderly, a meshed split-thickness skin graft is acceptable. In addition, a scrotal flap (modified Cecil technique) can be used to cover the denuded penis, as long as the patient does not mind a hair-bearing penis and is impotent.[12] To create the scrotal flap, a transverse incision is made in the inferior aspect of the scrotum followed by the formation of a subdartos tunnel. The penis is then mobilized through the tunnel, leaving only the glans exposed, while covering the denuded penile shaft. The scrotal flap edge is then sutured to the subcoronal skin

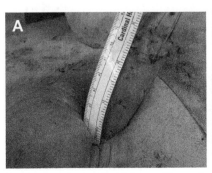 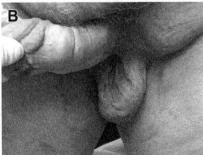

Fig. 6. (*A*) A thick nonmeshed split-thickness skin graft around the shaft of the penis. (*B*) Two months postoperative following penile skin grafting.

with interrupted absorbable sutures. Patients have the option to undergo a second-stage repair to free the penis, which few select.

PENILE FRACTURE

Fracture of the penis is a tear of the tunica albuginea of the corpus cavernosum, frequently while the penis is rigid and erect. When erect, the tunica albuginea stretches and thins to 0.25- to 0.5-mm-thick, compared with 2-mm-thick when flaccid.[17–20] Thus, the erect penis is more prone to serious injury (axial rupture) than the pendulous, flaccid penis during blunt trauma. In the Western Hemisphere, the most common cause of fracture is vigorous vaginal intercourse, most commonly when the woman is on top and the penis is acutely bent.[21,22] In the Middle East, however, the most common cause of fracture is self-penile manipulation in an attempt to achieve rapid detumescence.[23] Classically, signs and symptoms of penile fracture are a snapping or "popping" sound, followed by rapid detumescence, severe pain, ecchymosis, and swelling of the damaged side, with deviation away from the damaged side.[24,25] Typically, the penile fracture is a transverse corporal tear on the ventral portion of the penis, close to the urethra (**Fig. 8**). Many patients present in a delayed fashion because of embarrassment. The incidence of penile fracture is higher than prior reports, as some develop minor corporal tears, but never seek medical care.

Penile fracture is a clinical diagnosis. Imaging is not needed, particularly when the patient presents with a convincing history and physical examination.[12] Despite that there are numerous reports of the accuracy of cavernosography and magnetic resonance imaging to diagnose penile fractures, such methods are too invasive, time consuming, or costly to justify, particularly when the diagnosis can be made clinically.[19] Although sexual trauma

can also lead to the rupture of the dorsal vein of the penis and mimic penile fracture, the use of diagnostic imaging should be highly selective (**Fig. 9**). In contrast, if urethral injury is suspected, retrograde urethrography or flexible cystoscopy must be performed. Urethral injury has been reported in 10% to 38% of penile fracture cases.[1] Any signs of urethral injury, such as difficulty voiding, blood at the urethral meatus, or any degree of hematuria, should cause a high index of suspicion in the physician and deserve further evaluation.

Immediate surgical repair is the treatment of choice for penile fracture, as low complication rates and good outcomes have been reported by numerous centers.[12] Although conservative management may be an option in patients with minor tears of the tunica albuginea, most untreated fractures will develop delayed and persistent penile pain or curvature with erection. However, Kozacioglu and colleagues[26] have looked at delayed versus immediate repair and concluded that delayed repair had no ill effect as a consequence of a delay in surgery in patients without urethral involvement. Neither serious deformities nor erectile dysfunction was seen in the long term for these patients who had delayed repair. Although penile fracture is treated as a surgical emergency, from a practical view, waiting until the next morning for repair seems reasonable.

Surgical repair of the fracture requires exposure of the defect in the corpora cavernosum and gross inspection of the urethra, given the 20% rate of associated urethral injury.[12] Depending on the location of the injury, the options for exposure include a circumferential, subcoronal, degloving incision of the penile skin or a longitudinal incision directly over the injury exposing only the tunica tear. At first, the hematoma should be evacuated and the fracture site washed out. If the location of

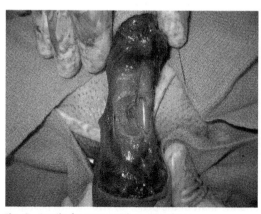

Fig. 8. Penile fracture with urethral tear.

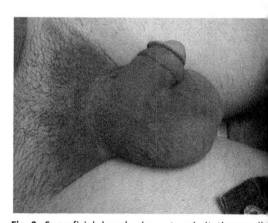

Fig. 9. Superficial dorsal vein rupture imitating penile fracture.

e corporal tear is not clear, a Penrose tourniquet
n be placed at the penile base with a butterfly
edle placed into the corporal shaft and injected
th saline (as in a Gittes test). Extravasating saline
ually helps identify the location of the defect. Pri-
ary closure of the corpora is usually performed
sing a running absorbable suture (2-0 Vicryl).

Complete urethral disruptions should be reanas-
mosed without delay, with the ends debrided,
atulated, and reapproximated tension-free
er a urethral catheter. If there is a partial tear
the urethra, then a "stenting" urethral catheter
n be placed with a suprapubic tube, but primary
pair of the tear should be performed when
ssible. Pericatheter urethrography is performed
ter 2 to 3 weeks after the procedure to confirm
ethral healing before catheter removal.

STICULAR RUPTURE

testicular rupture is a tear of the tunica albuginea
th extrusion of seminiferous tubules (**Fig. 10**).
though both penetrating and blunt mechanisms
n cause testicular rupture, most are blunt. The
je group most vulnerable to testicular rupture is
)- to –30-year-old men and boys involved in
orts-associated activity or motor vehicle acci-
ents.[27] In all cases of blunt scrotal trauma, the
hysician should have a high index of suspicion
d the rupture ruled out. Clinical examination
an be rather difficult in these patients because
any present with severe pain and swelling.

Although all penetrating injuries deep to the
crotal dartos fascia should be surgically
xplored, not all blunt injuries require exploration.
lany physicians will conservatively manage inries that do not show clinical or radiological

evidence of rupture. Scrotal ultrasonography, in
the hands of a skilled sonographer, can serve as
a vital addition to the physical examination, particularly if examination findings are equivocal.[28–31]
The sonographic findings are a heterogeneous
echo pattern of the testicular parenchyma with
loss of contour of the testis tunica (100% sensitivity and 93.5% specificity).[32] Injuries that are clinically benign and homogeneously echogenic on
ultrasound do not require surgical exploration.

In all cases of testicular rupture, urgent surgical
exploration is essential for salvage of the testicle.[12]
Although testis rupture is not life threatening, it can
have numerous repercussions including infertility,
hypogonadism, and low self-esteem. The surgeon
should attempt to salvage/preserve any remaining
viable tubules, as studies have revealed reduced
endocrine abnormalities and improved semen
quality compared with orchiectomy.[33,34] Blunt
ruptured testes explored within 72 hours have a
salvage rate of greater than 90%, whereas those
explored late have a 45% salvage rate.[35]

To achieve maximal exposure to both testes and
cords in addition to maintaining cosmesis, the
scrotum is typically explored through a vertical
incision of the median raphé. The tunica vaginalis
is then opened and the testis is brought out of
the scrotum and the testicle is inspected for injury.
Any nonviable seminiferous tubules are then
sharply excised and any hematoma is drained,
leaving only healthy bleeding edges. The tunica albuginea is then closed, using a running 3-0 absorbable suture (**Fig. 11**). The testis is returned into the
scrotum, with the lateral groove of the testis oriented properly to prevent torsion, and the scrotum
is closed in 2 layers with absorbable sutures. A
Penrose or closed suction drain can be placed
through a separate stab incision if hemostasis is
a concern. The wound is protected with fluff gauze

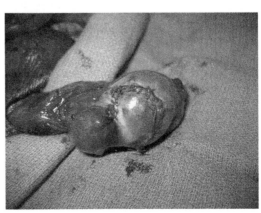

ig. 10. Close-up view of testis rupture with extrusion
f seminiferous tubules.

Fig. 11. Closure of tunica albuginea following testis
rupture.

and held in place with a scrotal support for compression. Anti-inflammatory medications, ice packs, and scrotal elevation may limit postoperative edema and hasten convalescence.

PENETRATING WOUNDS

Penetrating trauma to the genitalia is rare. Most cases are gunshot wounds (GSW) but stab wounds make up a significant portion. Although military GSW are from high-velocity weapons with significant injuries, most civilian GSW reported are from low-velocity weapons, causing less acute and delayed tissue damage.[36] All patients with penetrating penile wounds require a retrograde urethrography or urethroscopy, because up to 50% have an associated urethral injury.[37–39]

Early surgical exploration, debridement, and primary repair of penetrating injuries are the preferred management for both the penis and the testes.[40] Repair of a penetrating penile wound is comparable to that of a penile fracture. Depending on the location, direct visualization of the corpora can be obtained via a circumferential, degloving, subcoronal incision or via a penoscrotal, infrapubic, or perineal incision for more extensive wounds.[12] For minor injuries to the corpora, primary closure is adequate, as it is done for penile fractures.

Repair of testicular injury from a penetrating trauma also follows the same principles as that from a rupture from a blunt injury. Approximately 50% of GSW to the scrotum strike the testis and, of these, one-half of the testes are viable for repair.[12] Much like testicular rupture, salvage of viable testicular tissue is the primary goal of management. After debridement of the nonviable tissue, the tunica albuginea is closed primarily. In cases where the defect is wide and there is a deficiency of tunica albuginea to close primarily, a free graft of tunica vaginalis is used to cover the defect and preserve the testicle.[41] A tunica vaginalis graft can be easily harvested and sewn to the edges of the tunica albuginea for coverage (**Fig. 12**). Synthetic grafts (ie, Gore-Tex) result in poor outcomes secondary to infection and eventual orchiectomy. Thus, using the native tunica vaginalis tissue is the optimal tissue for coverage, and a clear alternative to orchiectomy.[12]

PENILE AMPUTATION

Traumatic genital amputations are usually self-mutilations performed by acutely psychotic patients or transsexuals unable to have (afford) sexual reassignment surgery.[42–47] A multidisciplinary team of urologists, plastic surgeons, psychiatrists, and social workers is needed to care

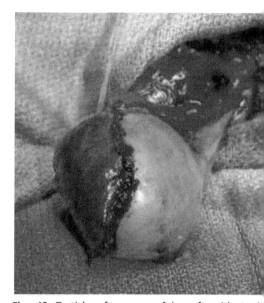

Fig. 12. Testicle after successful graft with tunic vaginalis.

for the penile amputation patient properly. Les commonly, genital amputations are caused b agricultural and industrial machinery accidents. Of note, the largest series of reanastamosis of penile amputations was reported in Thailand. During the 1970s, there were an estimated 10 penile amputations by angry wives against the philandering husbands, with 18 cases replante at the same medical center.

There are 3 options to treat the amputated peni depending on the degree of damage: closure of th residual stump, surgical reanastamosis of th amputated penis, or total phallic substitution wit reconstruction regardless of the psychologica state of the patient. Once the psychotic episod is properly treated, most patients are very remorse ful of self-amputation. If the amputated penis i viable, penile reanastamosis should always be a tempted. The amputated penis should be tho oughly washed out and debrided with eithe normal saline or lactated Ringer solution and the cooled in a "double bag."[50] The "double-bag technique involves wrapping the amputated peni in saline-soaked gauze and then placing it in a firs sterile sealed bag. Next, the first bag is placed in second bag or basin of ice-slush. This maneuve protects the penile skin from direct contact wit ice while still maintaining a hypothermic state, opt mally at 4°C. Penile replantation is attempted up t 24 hours after the injury because success has bee reported after 16 hours of cold ischemia an 6 hours of warm ischemia.[51,52]

The patient should be stabilized, with aggres sive fluid resuscitation and blood transfusio s indicated.[45] Whenever feasible, the patient should be cared for at a center that has the capability of performing microvascular surgery by a specialist.[44,46] Microvascular reattachment has shown superior outcomes with decreased skin necrosis and glans slough, improved sensation, and superior function when compared with macrovascular technique. If a patient cannot be treated at a center with microvascular capabilities, then a macrovascular reattachment can be attempted. This reattachmentn is certainly suboptimal, for the reasons stated above, but is a better option then defaulting to a penile stump.

To begin replantation, vascular control is obtained at the base of the proximal cut edge of the corpora. Local compression with gauze or tourniquet may be required depending on the extent of the hemorrhage. After controlled hemostasis, the tunica albuginea of the corpora cavernosa should be reapproximated with interrupted 3-0 polyglactin (Vicryl) suture. Placement of several sutures through the intercavernous septum will provide stabilization. The central cavernosal arteries do not need to be reanastamosed, because it does not improve outcome. The proximal and distal urethral edges are then mobilized for about 1 cm with the ends spatulated. Next, the urethra is reanastomosed over a 16-French silicone Foley catheter with interrupted 5-0 or 6-0 polydioxanone (Maxon, United States Surgical Corporation, Norwalk, CT, USA or PDS, Ethicon, Somerville, NJ, USA) suture in a single layer. Placement of a suprapubic tube is recommended to divert the urine proximally to facilitate healing.[12]

Once the penis is stabilized, then the deep dorsal vein is microscopically re-anastamosed with 11-0 nylon or polypropylene (Prolene, Ethicon, Somerville, NJ, USA). This anastamosis is critical and must be patent to prevent corporal edema, swelling, and subsequent ischemia. Next, at least one, preferably both, of the dorsal penile arteries are reapproximated in an end-to-end fashion, which immediately re-establishes blood flow to the subcutaneous tissues and prevents postoperative skin necrosis. Last, as many nerve fibers as can be identified are then reapproximated with a simple nylon or polypropylene suture in the epineurium. Dopplerable blood flow though the dorsal arteries needs to be confirmed before completing the case.[12]

If penile skin is intact, the skin edges are either reapproximated with interrupted 4-0 chromic sutures or a thick, nonmeshed, split-thickness skin graft is placed when the penile skin is unusable or denuded. A last resort and less attractive method of coverage is to bury the penis in a subcutaneous tunnel in the scrotum (using a modified Cecil technique), which leads to a suboptimal hair-bearing, thick-skinned penile shaft, which may require additional surgery.[10] It is crucial to cover the vascular anastamoses to avoid delayed thrombosis and necrosis and replantation failure. Finally, the penis is wrapped in loose dressings and an external splint is fashioned vertically to facilitate venous and lymphatic drainage.

If penile replantation is not an option because of loss of the detached penis or damaged beyond repair, then the penile stump can be closed as done for a standard elective partial penectomy (**Fig. 13**). The neomatus is widely spatulated to prevent stenosis. A free forearm phalloplasty can be performed subsequently.

Postoperative management must include at least 48 hours of bed rest and perioperative broad-spectrum antibiotics. The Foley catheter can be removed after at least 3 weeks of stenting, following a pericatheter retrograde urethrogram or a voiding cystourethrogram, which verifies a healed anastomosis. The suprapubic tube is capped and then removed after a few days of normal voiding. In cases of self-mutilation, the patient's mental health must be addressed and closely monitored and the psychiatry department must be involved with this patient's care.

TESTIS AMPUTATION

Although the penis, if properly cooled, can be successfully replanted, the testes are much more delicate and cannot tolerate extended periods of warm ischemia. Due to their highly metabolic state, the testes have only a 4- to 6-hour period following amputation for successful replantation.[10] If the patient is at risk for hypogonadal state, as with an atrophic or absent contralateral testis, microvascular technique is recommended for the best possible outcome.

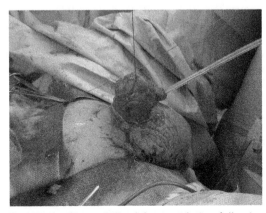

Fig. 13. Urethra mobilized for spatulation following penile amputation.

First, the 2 edges of the spermatic cord are debrided and the spermatic veins, the spermatic artery, and the vas deferens must be identified within both ends. The spermatic artery is anastamosed together using an 11-0 nylon or Prolene suture under microscopic view. If performed properly, the spermatic veins will begin to bleed on the testicular side and can be easily identified. If technically feasible, then at least 2 veins should be joined together with their severed counterparts. Last, the vas deferens must be realigned via a vasovasostomy in an end-to-end fashion performed in a 2-layer fashion, connecting first the vasal mucosa using 10-0 nylon or Prolene suture. The vasal muscularis is reapproximated using 9-0 nylon or Prolene suture, and then the spermatic fascia is closed primarily. To protect and support the fragile anastamoses, an orchiopexy is performed to secure the testicle in place. If the native scrotal skin is viable, the scrotum should be closed primarily over the reattached testis. Conversely, if more than 60% of the scrotal skin is absent, then the replanted testicles should be placed in thigh pouches until a neoscrotum is reconstructed, in the method described earlier for scrotal avulsion.

In all cases of self-inflicted genital amputation, patients must be closely observed following replantation surgery. Psychiatry must be closely engaged in these patients' care, because they are likely to repeat their actions if not properly managed.

MANAGEMENT OF COMPLEX UROLOGIC WOUNDS

Many traumatic wounds are difficult to manage despite optimal care. At times, the wound defect may be so large or complex that reconstruction is not feasible. Negative pressure wound therapy (NPWT) is not a new concept in wound therapy; it was first reported by Fleischmann and colleagues[53] in 1993. An NPWT device (VAC Therapy; Kinetic Concepts, Inc, San Antonio, TX, USA) is used to create a negative pressure over the wound, which drains the excessive interstitial edema, decompresses small vessels, and restores local blood flow. Other benefits of NPWT include reduction of bacterial colonization and stimulation granulation tissue growth to promote wound closure. To set up an NPWT, a piece of foam is placed over the wound with a large piece of transparent tape cover and a drain tube is set to transport fluid to a vacuum pump. Any open wound can be converted into a controlled closed wound with an NPWT device.

An NPWT may be used for many types of wounds, including dehisced surgical wounds, complex operative wounds left open to heal by secondary intention, meshed skin grafts and flaps, stage III and IV pressure ulcers, chronic open wounds, diabetic foot ulcers, venous stasis ulcers, degloving injuries, and partial-thickness and full thickness burns (<12 hours of burn). It should not be used for patients with malignancy, necrotic tissue that has not been debrided, fistulae to body cavities/organs, untreated osteomyelitis, wounds with bleeding bed, or patients on anticoagulation therapy.[54]

In 2005, Armstrong and colleagues[55] enrolled 162 patients with complex wounds after a partial foot amputation into a 16-week, multicenter, randomized, clinical trial. Seventy-seven patients were randomly assigned to NPWT with dressing changes every 48 hours versus 85 control patients who received standard moist wound care according to consensus guidelines. NPWT was delivered through the vacuum-assisted closure therapy system. Wounds were treated until healing or completion of the 112-day period of active treatment. This study showed that the NPWT group healed more than the control group (43 [56%] vs 33 [39%], $P = .040$). The time to complete wound closure was also faster in the NPWT group than in controls ($P = .005$). In addition, the rate of granulation tissue formation was faster in the NPWT group than in controls ($P = .002$).

The costs of NPWT are significant, and this has discouraged many clinicians from using the therapy. However, there are reports showing the faster healing time with NPWT compared with conventional therapies correlating to decreased overall cost of care.[56] Philbeck and colleagues showed that the average wound closure rate with an NPWT (vacuum-assisted closure) was 0.23 cm^2/d compared with 0.09 cm^2/d for a wound treated with saline-soaked gauze. The average 22.2-cm^2 wound in the study took 247 days to heal at a cost of $23,465 with saline-soaked gauze versus 97 days to heal at a cost of $14,546 with an NPWT system. The study showed that the NPWT is an efficacious and economical therapy option for variety of chronic wounds.

NPWT combines the benefit of both open-wound and closed-wound treatment. NPWT is not universally applicable to all type of wounds however. In a carefully selected patient, it can serve as a practical addition to the traditional wound therapy options available to the reconstructive surgeon.

SUMMARY

Traumatic genital injury predominantly affects the young and is usually not life threatening evertheless, the treating physician must have a gh index of suspicion when evaluating genital injuries. Although missed diagnosis can result in re consequence with life-long sequelae, rapid nd proper treatment can help preserve tissue, osmesis, and function.

EFERENCES

1. Brandes SB, McAninch JW. External genital trauma: amputation, degloving, and burns. Atlas Urol Clin 1998;6:127–42.
2. McDougal WS, Peterson HD, Pruitt BA, et al. The thermally injured perineum. J Urol 1997;121:320–4.
3. Peck MD, Boileau MA, Grube BJ, et al. The management of burns to the perineum and genitals. J Burn Care Rehabil 1990;11:54–6.
4. Michielsen D, Van Hee R, Neetens C, et al. Burns to genitalia and the perineum. J Urol 1998;159:418–9.
5. Evers LH, Bhavsar D, Mailänder P. The biology of burn injury. Exp Dermatol 2010;19(9):777–83.
6. Morey AF, Metro MJ, Carney KJ, et al. Consensus on genitourinary trauma: external genitalia. BJU Int 2004;94:507–15.
7. Gomes CM, Ribeiro-Filho L, Giron AM, et al. Genital trauma due to animal bites. J Urol 2000;165:80–3.
8. Talan DA, Citron DM, Abrahamian FM, et al. Bacteriologic analysis of infected dog and cat bites. N Engl J Med 1999;340:85–92.
9. Talan DA, Abrahamian FM, Moran GJ, et al. Clinical presentation and bacteriologic analysis of infected human bites in patients presenting to emergency departments. Clin Infect Dis 2003;37(11):1481–9.
10. Armenakas NA, McAninch JW. Genital reconstruction after major skin loss. In: McAninch JW, editor. Traumatic and reconstructive urology. Philadelphia: WB Saunders; 1996. p. 699–713.
11. McAninch JW. Management of genital skin loss. Urol Clin North Am 1989;16:387–97.
12. Ferguson GG, Brandes S. Reconstruction for genital trauma. In: Montague D, editor. Textbook of reconstructive urologic surgery. London: Informa; 2008. p. 657–67.
13. Balakrishnan C. Scrotal avulsion: a new technique of reconstruction by split-skin graft. Br J Plast Surg 1956;9:38–42.
14. Wessells H, Long L. Penile and genital injuries. Urol Clin North Am 2006;33:117–26.
15. Cummings JM, Boullier JA. Scrotal dog bites. J Urol 2000;164(1):57–8.
16. Morey AF, Dugi D. Genital and lower urinary tract trauma. In: Wein A, editor. Campbell-Walsh urology. Philadelphia: Elsevier Saunders; 2012. p. 2507–13.
17. Fetter TR, Gartman E. Traumatic rupture of the penis. Am J Surg 1936;32:371–2.
18. Thompson RF. Rupture of the penis. J Urol 1954;71: 226–9.
19. Choi MH, Kim B, Ryu JA, et al. MR imaging of acute penile fracture. Radiographics 2000;20:1397–405.
20. Miller S, McAninch JW. Penile fracture and soft tissue injury. In: McAninch JW, editor. Traumatic and reconstructive urology. Philadelphia: WB Saunders; 1996. p. 693–8.
21. Mydlo JH. Surgeon experience with penile fracture. J Urol 2001;166:526–9.
22. Eke N. Fracture of the penis. Br J Surg 2002;89: 555–65.
23. Zargooshi J. Penile fracture in Kermanshah, Iran: report of 172 cases. J Urol 2000;164:364–6.
24. El-Taher AM, Aboul-Ella HA, Sayed MA, et al. Management of penile fracture. J Trauma 2004;56: 1138–40.
25. Beysel M, Tekin A, Gurdal M, et al. Evaluation and treatment of penile fractures: accuracy of clinical diagnosis and the value of corpus cavernosography. Urology 2002;60:492–6.
26. Kozacioglu Z, Degirmenci T, Arslan M, et al. Long-term significance of the number of hours until surgical repair of penile fractures. Urol Int 2011;87:75–9.
27. Baskin LS, McAninch JW. Reconstruction of testicular rupture. In: McAninch JW, editor. Traumatic and reconstructive urology. Philadelphia: WB Saunders; 1996. p. 693–8.
28. Corrales JG, Corbel L, Cipolla B, et al. Accuracy of ultrasound diagnosis after blunt testicular trauma. J Urol 1993;150:1834–6.
29. Ugarte R, Spaedy M, Cass AS. Accuracy of ultrasound in diagnosis of rupture after blunt testicular trauma. Urology 1990;36:253–4.
30. Anderson KA, McAninch JW, Jeffrey RB, et al. Ultrasonography for the diagnosis and staging of blunt scrotal trauma. J Urol 1983;130:933–5.
31. Fournier GR Jr, Laing FC, Jeffrey RB, et al. High resolution scrotal ultrasonography: a highly sensitive but nonspecific diagnostic technique. J Urol 1985;134:490–3.
32. Buckley JC, McAninch JW. Diagnosis and management of testicular ruptures. Urol Clin North Am 2006;33:111–6.
33. Lin WW, Kim ED, Quesada ET, et al. Unilateral testicular injury from external trauma: evaluation of semen quality and endocrine parameters. J Urol 1998;159:841–3.
34. Kukadia AN, Ercole CJ, Gleich P, et al. Testicular trauma: potential impact on reproductive function. J Urol 1996;156:1643–6.
35. Cass AS. Testicular trauma. J Urol 1983;129: 299–300.
36. Brandes SB, Buckman RF, Chelsky MJ, et al. External genitalia gunshot wounds: a ten-year experience with 56 cases. J Trauma 1995;39:266–72.

37. Miles BJ, Poffenberger RJ, Farah RN, et al. Management of penile gunshot wounds. Urology 1990;36:318–21.

38. Monga M, Moreno T, Hellstrom WJ. Gunshot wounds to the male genitalia. J Trauma 1995;38:855–8.

39. Cline KJ, Mata JA, Venable DD, et al. Penetrating trauma to the male external genitalia. J Trauma 1998;44:492–4.

40. Bandi G, Santucci RA. Controversies in the management of male external genitourinary trauma. J Trauma 2004;56:1362–70.

41. Ferguson GG, Brandes SB. Gunshot wound injury of the testis: the use of tunica vaginalis and polytetrafluoroethylene grafts for reconstruction. J Urol 2007;178:2462–5.

42. Baltieri DA, Guerra de Andrade A. Transsexual self-mutilation. Am J Forensic Med Pathol 2005;26:268–70.

43. Greilsheimer H, Groves JE. Male genital self-mutilation. Arch Gen Psychiatry 1979;36:441–6.

44. Aboseif S, Gomez R, McAninch JW. Genital self-mutilation. J Urol 1993;150:1143–6.

45. Mora W, Drach GW. Self emasculation and self castration: immediate surgical management and ultimate psychological adjustment. J Urol 1980;124:208–9.

46. Jezior JR, Brady JD, Schlossberg SM. Management of penile amputation injuries. World J Surg 2001;25:1602–9.

47. Darewicz B, Galek L, Darewicz J, et al. Successful microsurgical replantation of an amputated penis. Int Urol Nephrol 2001;33:385–6.

48. Dogra PN, Gautam G, Ansari MS. Penile amputation and emasculation: hazards of modern agricultural machinery. Int Urol Nephrol 2004;36:379–80.

49. Bhanganada K, Chayavatana T, Pongnumkul C, et al. Surgical management of an epidemic of penile amputations in Siam. Am J Surg 1983;146:376–82.

50. Jordan GH. Initial management and reconstruction of male genital amputation injuries. In: McAninch JW, editor. Traumatic and reconstructive urology. Philadelphia: WB Saunders; 1996. p. 673–81.

51. Wei FC, McKee NH, Huerta FJ, et al. Microsurgic replantation of a completely amputated penis. Ann Plast Surg 1983;20:317–21.

52. Hayhurst SW, O'Brien BM, Ishida H. Experimental digital replantation after prolonged cooling. Hand 1974;6:134–41.

53. Fleischmann W, Strecker W, Bombelli M, et al. Vacuum sealing as treatment of soft tissue damage in open fractures. Unfallchirurg 1993;96(9):488–92.

54. Health Quality Ontario. Negative pressure wound therapy: an evidence based analysis. Ont Health Technol Assess Ser 2006;6(14):1–83.

55. Armstrong DG, Lavery LA, Diabetic Foot Study Consortium. Negative pressure wound therapy after partial diabetic foot amputation: a multicentre randomised controlled trial. Lancet 2005;366(9498):1704–10.

56. Philbeck TE Jr, Whittington KT, Millsap MH, et al. The clinical and cost effectiveness of externally applied negative pressure wound therapy in the treatment of wounds in home healthcare Medicare patients. Ostomy Wound Manage 1999;45:41–50.

Skin Grafting of the Penis

Hema J. Thakar, MD[a], Daniel D. Dugi III, MD[b],*

KEYWORDS

- Penile reconstruction • Skin grafting • Penile lymphedema • Penile trauma • Fournier gangrene

KEY POINTS

- Choice of reconstruction of penile skin loss depends on anatomic and functional factors.
- Normal skin graft healing involves imbibition, inosculation, and revascularization.
- The most common causes of skin graft loss are hematoma, seroma, infection, or shear.
- Skin grafting of the penis can be challenging because of the ability of the penis to change size.

INTRODUCTION

Penile skin loss may occur after a variety of disease processes. Reconstructive options are tailored to the defect. When skin is missing, skin grafting can achieve the goal of reconstructing like with like.

Even urologists who do not specialize in reconstruction may be called on to give their advice in complex cases, especially after necrotizing genital infections. Although they are experts in general reconstructive principles, plastic surgeons may not be aware of the unique anatomic and functional factors in penile and genital reconstruction; collaborative efforts are often necessary.

INDICATIONS FOR PENILE SKIN GRAFTING

Several disease processes may cause actual or functional loss of penile skin, and skin grafting is often necessary to reconstruct these wounds. The most common problems include necrotizing infections of genital skin (ie, Fournier gangrene), lichen sclerosus, trauma, and burns. Resection of penile cancer or genital lymphedema may require removal of skin from the penis, leading to a need for replacement. A circumcision sometimes results in too much skin removal and the need for a skin graft. In addition, reoperative repair of hypospadias or penile urethral stricture may use oral mucosal or skin grafting.

SKIN ANATOMY

Skin has many roles, most importantly serving as a barrier to the outside world. The skin has 3 layers: the epidermis, the dermis, and the hypodermis or subcutaneous layer (**Fig. 1**). The epidermis, the most superficial layer, produces and maintains the stratum corneum, the waterproof outermost barrier of the skin. The epidermis also contains important specialized cells such as melanocytes, immune cells, and sensory cells.

The dermis makes up the remaining 90% to 95% of the total skin thickness and provides a collagen matrix to support the epidermis. The skin appendages, such as hair follicles, sweat glands, and sebaceous glands are found in the dermis. The hair follicle has multipotent bulb cells that are important in reepithelialization of a wound.[1,2]

TERMINOLOGY

A skin graft is skin that is removed from one anatomic location, without a blood supply, and

Funding Sources: None.
Conflict of Interest: None.
[a] Division of Plastic and Reconstructive Surgery, Department of Surgery, Oregon Health and Sciences University, Mail Code: CH5P, 3303 Southwest Bond Avenue, Portland, OR 97239, USA; [b] Department of Urology, Oregon Health and Sciences University, Mail Code: CH10U, 3303 Southwest Bond Avenue, Portland, OR 97239, USA
* Corresponding author.
E-mail address: dugi@ohsu.edu

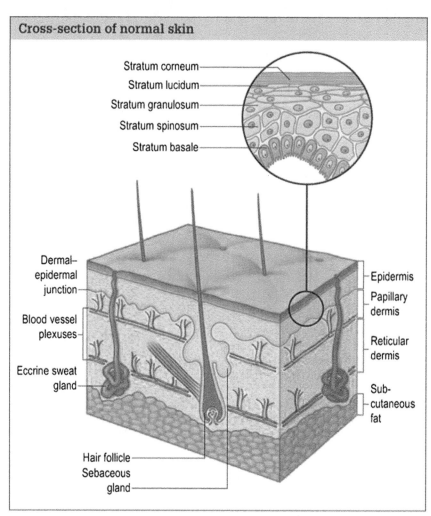

Fig. 1. Layers of the skin. (*From* Fang RC, Mustoe TA. Structure and function of the skin. In: Guyuron B, Eriksson E Persing JA, editors. Plastic surgery: indications and practice. Philadelphia: Saunders Elsevier; 2009; with permission.)

transplanted to a new site. Engraftment is the process of revascularization and healing of the graft. Skin grafts are commonly categorized in terms of the depth of the graft. A full-thickness skin graft is comprised of all the dermis and epidermis. This graft is harvested at the interface of the dermis and hypodermis (see **Fig. 1**). The thickness of this graft is determined by the anatomic site from which is it is harvested. For example, a full-thickness skin graft obtained from the prepuce is thinner than a graft harvested from the back. In the case of a full-thickness skin graft, the donor site is closed primarily. In contrast, a split-thickness skin graft comprises the epidermis and only a portion of the dermis. It is harvested with a dermatome, an instrument that shaves a sheet of skin of controlled width and thickness.

DIFFERENCES BETWEEN SPLIT-THICKNESS AND FULL-THICKNESS SKIN GRAFTS

There is more dermis in a full-thickness skin graft than in a split-thickness skin graft, so there are some important distinctions in the behavior and potential use of both types of grafts (**Table 1**). Because split-thickness skin grafts are thinner and have less tissue, they have less metabolic demand from the wound bed, and thus have better survival or take. In contrast, a full-thickness skin graft is thicker and, as such, has greater metabolic demand. Survival of a full-thickness skin graft is more uncertain and it requires a well-vascularized recipient site.

Full-thickness skin grafts display significantly more primary contraction than split-thickness

Table 1
Characteristics of full-thickness and split-thickness skin grafts

	Full-thickness Skin Graft	Split-thickness Skin Graft
Amount of dermis	More	Less
Primary contracture	More	Less
Secondary contracture	Less	More
Metabolic activity	More	Less
Hair growth	More	Less
Sweat gland function	More	Less
Sebaceous gland function	More	Less
Sensory return	More	Less

skin grafts. Primary contraction is the recoil that occurs immediately after a skin graft is harvested and is directly related to the amount of elastin present in the dermis. A full-thickness skin graft can lose up to 40% of its surface area from primary contraction. These rates are lower with grafts that have less dermis. For example, a thin split-thickness skin graft only loses 10% of its surface area from primary contraction.[3]

Over time, full-thickness skin grafts have a tendency to resist the significant problem of secondary contraction, the contraction of a skin graft after healing. Myofibroblasts within the graft are primarily responsible for secondary contraction. The use of thicker skin grafts, with more dermis, helps to prevent this type of contraction. Once secondary contraction ends, full-thickness skin grafts tend to stretch and grow with an individual, whereas split-thickness skin grafts tend not to expand as well.[3]

Another important distinction between full-thickness skin grafts and split-thickness skin grafts is the durability of the graft. Once again, this difference is directly related to the thickness of the dermal layer. Thicker grafts are better able to resist friction and trauma.

It is also notable that the skin's appendages, such as sweat and sebaceous glands, are present in the dermis. As such, full-thickness skin grafts have a greater ability to sweat or produce oil. However, this ability depends on the reinnervation of the glands, which can take several months to years. In the interim, it is important to keep skin grafts well moisturized to prevent drying, which can lead to fissuring of the grafted skin, especially for split-thickness skin grafts, which are lacking in these glands permanently.

Hair follicles are also present in the dermis, and full-thickness skin grafts show the hair growth pattern of the donor site. It is therefore important to make sure that full-thickness skin grafts used in penile reconstruction are obtained from a hairless area. Split-thickness skin grafts are generally hairless and thus are preferred on the penis.

In choosing a skin graft, donor site morbidity must also be considered. A full-thickness graft, by definition, leaves a full-thickness defect at the donor site, and large donor sites may be difficult to close or hide. Split-thickness grafts have the benefit of leaving a donor site that heals with only simple wound care. In addition, the thickness of dermis varies by anatomic site and with age. The dermis is thinner in children and with advancing age,[4] and what may be a thick split-thickness graft in a young adult patient may leave a full-thickness wound in the elderly.

CHOICE OF SKIN GRAFT IN PENILE RECONSTRUCTION

The choice of graft thickness depends on the needs of the wound to be covered and the inherent compromises associated with graft thickness. A core principle of reconstructing tissue loss is to replace like with like, meaning choosing donor tissue that most closely replicates the native tissue in function and appearance. The skin of the penis is thin, hairless, and flexible. Because of the dramatic change in size of the penis with erection and the need for durability because of the tissue demands of sexual activity, full-thickness skin grafts seem to be the preferred choice in the replacement of penile skin. Although some prefer full-thickness grafts in penile skin replacement,[5] in most cases it is best replaced by a split-thickness skin graft (**Fig. 2**).[6,7] A thick split-thickness skin graft offers the best combination of graft take and durability.

In some cases, a full-thickness skin graft may be appropriate in penile reconstruction. The most common example is in urethral reconstruction. Although a detailed discussion of graft urethroplasty is outside the scope of this review, understanding the principles behind graft selection and the factors that determine success is essential. Urethral reconstruction calls for tissue that resists the stress of urine passage. At present, a full-thickness oral mucosal graft is the closest replacement tissue for the urethra. It is used extensively in staged reconstruction of urethral repairs and

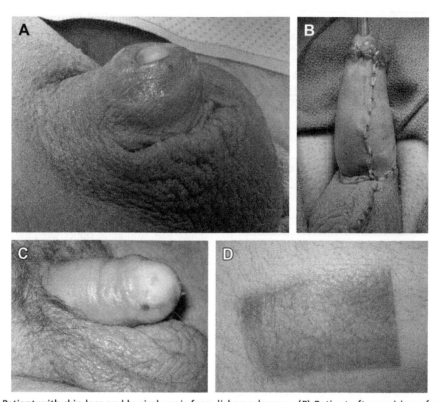

Fig. 2. (A) Patient with skin loss and buried penis from lichen sclerosus. (B) Patient after excision of scarred ski and split-thickness skin grafting to penis. (C) Patient 5 weeks after surgery. (D) Lateral thigh skin graft donor sit 5 weeks after surgery.

complex hypospadias.[8] Meshed foreskin and split-thickness skin grafts used in staged urethral reconstruction[9] have fallen from favor, especially as oral mucosal grafts have come into use. In some circumstances, the prepuce of an uncircumcised patient may be used to reconstruct penile skin elsewhere.

NORMAL SKIN GRAFT HEALING

Engraftment involves removing tissue (skin or mucosa) from its native location and blood supply and transferring it to a recipient bed, where the transplanted tissue undergoes revascularization. Disruption of this process leads to graft failure.

The first phase of engraftment is known as plasmatic imbibition and lasts for 24 to 48 hours. During this time, the diffusion of nutrients, oxygen, and metabolic waste occurs passively back and forth across the concentration gradient from the graft to the wound bed.[10] For the duration of the imbibition phase, the graft is without blood flow and appears white. Greater vascularity of the wound bed results in shorter graft ischemia time. Because it is composed of more tissue and has

greater metabolic demand, a full-thickness ski graft can only tolerate this ischemia for abou 3 days. However, a split-thickness skin graft i more forgiving because it has less metabolic de mand. It can survive ischemia through imbibitio for up to 5 days.[11]

The next stage, inosculation, begins withi 36 hours and involves the formation of anastomoti connections between host and graft vasculature Skin grafts begin to have capillary refill during thi phase. As blood flow begins, it is disorganized a first. As such, especially full-thickness skin graft may appear slightly cyanotic at this time.[12]

During the final phase of skin graft healing revascularization, new vessels within the gra establish the definitive vasculature that will ensur the long-term survival of the graft. Whether th preexisting vessels in the graft act as conduit for ingrowth and become reendothelialized, o entirely new vessels form, or all of these occur, re mains an area of ongoing research.[13]

Over time, it is normal for skin grafts to becom hyperpigmented or hypopigmented. Grafts tha are harvested from the lower trunk and thigh have a tendency to darken or take on a yellov olor as the graft matures, especially with skin rafts from the groin. Thinner skin grafts have a greater tendency to be hyperpigmented.[14,15]

Skin grafts can reinnervate over time. The process of nerve ingrowth begins both from the wound bed and from the periphery of the skin graft, progressing inwards.[16] This process can take more than 2 years. The extent of reinnervation depends on the presence of neurilemmal sheaths within the graft. The more dermis that is present in the graft, the better the likelihood of reinnervation. Thus, full-thickness skin grafts have better potential for reinnervation than thin split-thickness skin grafts.[16]

ABNORMAL SKIN GRAFT HEALING

Adverse local factors and errors in surgical technique can lead to graft failure. The most common cause of graft failure is fluid accumulation under the graft. Hematoma or seroma formation between the graft and recipient bed increases the distance required for diffusion of nutrients during the imbibition phase. In addition, a hematoma can create a barrier between the graft and the wound bed, inhibiting revascularization.[17] Careful hemostasis is important to prevent this complication.

The second most common cause of skin graft failure is infection. Atraumatic graft handling and a well-vascularized and clean wound bed are paramount. Skin graft survival is improved when there are fewer than 10^5 colony-forming units of bacteria per gram of tissue.[18] Fibrin has a bacteriostatic effect and has an important role in the survival of skin grafts.[19]

Additional causes of graft failure include moving of the graft, or shearing. Shearing disrupts the neovascularization from the host bed to the graft. Quilting sutures may be placed to decrease the dead space between the graft and the recipient bed and to decrease shear injury.[17] The graft will fail any place where the graft is not in direct contact with the wound bed. Bolster or negative-pressure wound dressings can also help in this regard by helping to hold the graft in place on the wound bed.

TECHNIQUE OF SPLIT-THICKNESS SKIN GRAFTING

The first step in reconstruction after penile skin loss is preparing the wound bed. In cases of necrotizing genital infections, debridement of all necrotic tissues may take one or many surgical procedures. Once the wound bed is healthy, and the patient has been stabilized, reconstruction of the wound can proceed. Broad-spectrum antibiotics are administered before surgery. A urinary catheter is placed. The penile shaft and tunica vaginalis are good recipient graft beds, and the presence of granulation tissue is not necessary for skin graft coverage. The wound bed is debrided to decrease bacterial contamination.

Thick split-thickness skin grafts are preferred for replacement of the penile shaft skin. The dimensions of a wound may not be apparent until the penis is put on stretch or an erection is induced. At the least, the penis should be placed on stretch through the use of a glans suture when measuring to determine the necessary skin graft. Because of primary contraction, the size of the graft taken should be larger than the penile defect by approximately 20%. A split-thickness graft harvested for coverage of most locations may typically be 0.03 mm (0.0012 inch). For the penis, a thicker graft of 0.04 mm (0.0016 inch), with its associated greater amount of dermis, is better able to resist the friction and wear of sexual activity, and is elastic enough to stretch with erections.

The hair over the donor site is removed. The lateral thigh is generally used as a donor site because it can easily be draped within the area of the wound, and it is easy to procure a wide (75–100 mm [3–4 inch]) sheet graft from this area. In addition, compared with the medial thigh, the lateral thigh is less sensitive. The patient is asked before surgery regarding his preference as to which side to use, in an attempt to avoid harvesting from the side on which the patient sleeps. If the lateral thigh cannot be used, the abdominal wall, buttocks, or back can make suitable, but less convenient, donor sites. Some investigators advocate harvesting a split-thickness graft from the skin resected when treating genital lymphedema[20]; however, when skin is grossly abnormal it should be discarded.

The donor site is lubricated. Mineral oil is often used, but we prefer the use of chlorhexidine gluconate solution 4.0% because it is easier to remove and does not interfere with adhesive dressings. The donor skin is made taught with the aid of an assistant to help in procuring the graft. Next, the skin graft is obtained with a pneumatic or electric dermatome, such as a Zimmer (Zimmer, Warsaw, IN) or Padgett dermatome (Integra, Plainsboro, NJ). The donor site is then temporarily dressed with Telfa gauze (Covidien, Mansfield, MA) soaked in saline with epinephrine to help with hemostasis. A local anesthetic is injected to help with postoperative pain because the donor site is especially uncomfortable.

Creating an outlet for the egress of fluid is important in preventing hematomas or seromas. Meshing is a technique for providing drainage from beneath the graft. The graft is passed through a mesher on a plastic carrier that determines the expansion ratio. We typically mesh and expand grafts to the scrotum by 1:1.5. Meshing has the added benefit of allowing the graft to cover a greater surface area (**Fig. 3**). However, expanded meshed grafts yield a netlike scar pattern on healing. In addition, because the interstices heal by secondary intention, there is more contraction of the graft.

In cosmetically sensitive areas and where minimal graft contraction is desired, such as the penis, a nonmeshed graft, or sheet graft, is preferred. Instead of meshing, the pie-crusting technique (**Fig. 4**) allows fluid to drain from beneath a graft. This technique entails creating perforations in the graft with a blade. The perforations are oriented in a random pattern to avoid drawing the eye to any specific pattern.

The skin graft ideally is placed over the penile shaft in such a way that the incision line recreates the median raphe on the ventral surface (**Fig. 5**). The skin graft is sutured to the surrounding skin with 4-0 chromic sutures. Quilting sutures, placed in a manner avoiding the urethra and dorsal neurovascular bundle, should be used to adhere the graft closely to the wound bed to prevent seroma or shear. If the glans has been deepithelialized, as may be the case in patients with lichen sclerosus, skin graft is placed over the denuded area.

Fibrin glue has been shown to slightly improve skin graft take in simple reconstructions. However,

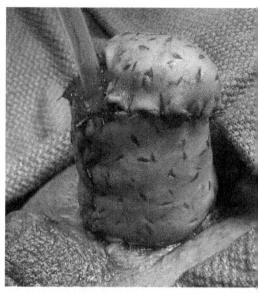

Fig. 4. A patient who had traumatic partial penil amputation and loss of penile skin underwent split thickness skin grafting with pie-crusting incisions o graft to allow for drainage of blood and serum fror beneath the graft.

its real benefit is in difficult areas to graft, such a the penis or perineum. Several studies have foun significant improvement in graft take when used i mobile areas or areas close to skin folds.[21,2 Using a thin layer of diluted fibrin glue may hel with graft adhesion[23] and minimize the concer of adding a barrier to imbibition and inosculation

Often the testes need skin coverage at the sam time as the penis, particularly after necrotizing genital infections or lymphedema. The scrotun may be reconstructed with thigh flaps, but w find split-thickness skin grafting of the scrotun to be less morbid and to heal with good cosmeti results, especially when the tunica vaginalis ha been preserved. The testes are sutured to on another in the midline. The skin graft is generall taken at 0.03 mm (0.0012 inch) thickness anc then meshed in a 1:1.5 ratio (see **Figs. 3** and 5B) The graft is then sutured to the tunica vaginali or directly to the tunica albuginea of the teste with 4-0 chromic sutures.

In cases in which only a small area of the peni requires grafting, such as in staged urethral recon struction, a tie-over bolster dressing is a simple efficient way of compressing the graft to preven hematoma or shear. Our preference is to use ster ile surgical prep sponges as the bolster on top o petrolatum gauze (**Fig. 6**). Sutures are placec through the adjacent penile skin and tied togethe over the bolster. The ties should be snug but not so tight as to damage the skin through which the

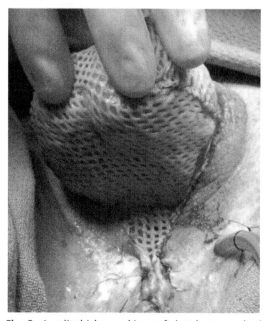

Fig. 3. A split-thickness skin graft has been meshed 1:1.5 and applied to the testicles and perineum.

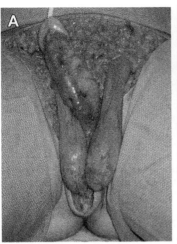
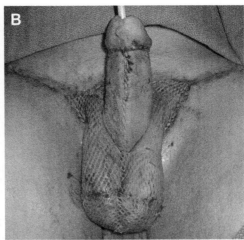

g. 5. (*A*) Perineal and penile wound after debridement of genital lymphedema. (*B*) Split-thickness skin grafting the perineum and penis. Note that the penile skin graft has been applied as a sheet graft and has been pie usted, whereas the perineal skin graft has been applied as a meshed graft. Some portions of the wound ve been repaired by primary closure.

uture is placed. A tie-over bolster may even be sed in glans reconstruction.[24]

For circumferential penile skin grafting, our preference is to dress the skin grafted areas with etrolatum gauze and a negative-pressure wound ressing.[25] Negative-pressure wound dressings uch as VAC Therapy, Kinetic Concepts, Inc, an Antonio, TX), may help the graft to conform osely to the underlying tissue, thus precluding e accumulation of fluid (**Fig. 7**A).[26] Circumferenal negative-pressure dressings on the penis have een shown to be safe and effective in penile skin rafting.[27] When applying a negative-pressure ound dressing to the penile shaft, we also apply ngue depressors outside the sponge to help aintain the length of the penis (see **Fig. 7**B), ecause the negative-pressure dressing will otherise not keep the penis stretched to length. The egative-pressure wound dressing is then placed 100 to 125 mm Hg continuous pressure. However, the negative-pressure dressing alone cannot e relied on to achieve contact between the graft

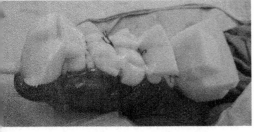

g. 6. A tie-over bolster is used to dress a full-hickness graft in staged urethral reconstruction.

and the bed, and areas of the graft that are not in direct contact with the recipient bed will necrose.

The dressing and urinary catheter are then left in place for 5 days, during which time the patient is kept on bed rest. After the dressing is removed, antibiotic ointment and petrolatum gauze are used to dress the wound until it has finished healing for the next 2 weeks. After this, the patient is instructed to apply lotion to the grafted areas daily as all skin grafts are without sebaceous gland activity, at least in the early healing period.

The skin graft donor site is covered with a semiocclusive dressing such as Tegaderm (3M, St Paul, Minnesota) or Op-Site (Smith & Nephew, St Petersburg, FL). Semiocclusive dressings tend to be more comfortable than leaving the wound open or using semiopen dressings such as scarlet red or petrolatum gauze.[28] The donor site may collect serous fluid while covered with a semiocclusive dressing. This fluid can be aspirated using sterile technique, and the puncture site covered with another semiocclusive dressing. If the donor site dressing is leaking, it can be reinforced or removed and petrolatum gauze placed over the donor site. Depending on the thickness of the skin graft, the donor site can take between 7 and 21 days to reepithelialize. Once the donor site has healed, the dressing is removed, and the patient is encouraged to apply lotion to the wound daily.

FULL-THICKNESS SKIN GRAFTING IN PENILE RECONSTRUCTION

Oral mucosal grafts are most often used full-thickness skin graft in genital reconstruction and

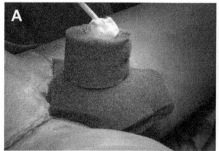
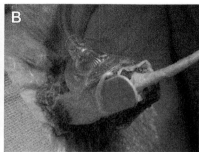

Fig. 7. (*A*) Negative-pressure wound sponge is placed over the skin graft as a bolster. (*B*) Negative-pressu⃓ wound dressing applied with tongue depressors cut to size outside the sponge to keep the penis to length.

are largely beyond the scope of this discussion. However, the use of full-thickness grafts in staged urethral reconstruction follows the same principles critical for success of split-thickness grafts: careful hemostasis, close apposition to the graft bed, and graft immobilization. Other sources of hairless skin may include abdominal or flank skin in some patients, supraclavicular skin, and postauricular skin. These grafts must be fully defatted to maximize their potential for engraftment. Although usually abundant, scrotal skin is typically not the best choice for penile skin replacement because it is hair bearing.

When harvesting a full-thickness skin graft, the target area is marked. Marking an ellipse 3 times as long as it is wide that includes the target area allows for primary wound closure without lateral wound redundancy. Once harvested, the graft should be defatted so that the dermis is in direct contact with the wound bed. This defatting may be done during the graft harvest, leaving the fat behind as the graft is harvested. As an alternative, the graft may be defatted on the back table. The authors prefer to do this with the graft draped over the surgeon's nondominant index finger, using sharp scissors on the convex surface of the graft (**Fig. 8**).

TIPS IN PENILE SKIN GRAFTING

Surgeons reconstructing penile skin loss after trauma or necrotizing infections must work with what tissue remains; often this means loss of tissue down to the Buck fascia. However, in elective circumstances, such as buried penis caused by lichen sclerosus or genital lymphedema, the surgeon must choose what tissue to resect, and this affects the outcome of the reconstruction. In the resection of penile lymphedema, the skin and dartos layer are removed down to the Buck fascia to prevent recurrence of lymphedema.[6] In other circumstances, such as surgery for lichen sclerosus, cicatricial and abnormal skin should

be resected leaving the underlying dartos tissu⃓ Because the dartos layer and loose tissue benea⃓ the skin are not tightly affixed to the Buck fasci⃓ grafting on the dartos layer preserves the skin mobility.

When there is loss of the proximal penile ski⃓ the natural tendency is to preserve any viab⃓ distal skin. However, when there is loss of th⃓ proximal penile skin, the proximal dartos layer generally also lost. This loss results in disruptic⃓ of lymphatic drainage of the distal penile ski⃓ The native skin should be resected to the level ⃓ the glans to avoid a ring of lymphedematous sk⃓ around the glans (**Fig. 9**). If skin loss is not circu⃓ ferential, it may be preferable to leave the nativ⃓ skin in place, especially if several days of observa⃓ tion have not led to increasing edema of the ski⃓

The glans penis is a unique structure where th⃓ skin layer is directly attached to the tunica albug⃓ nea beneath it. There are few situations in whic⃓ there is loss of skin of the glans without loss ⃓ the underlying spongy tissue. Because the peni⃓ shaft skin and glans have separate blood supplie⃓ most cases of penile skin loss do not invol⃓

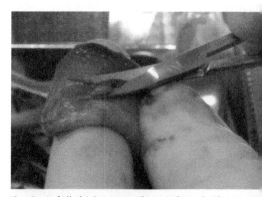

Fig. 8. A full-thickness graft is defatted. The conve⃓ surface of the finger and the oppositely convex curv⃓ of the scissors allows precision in where the hypode⃓ mis is excised.

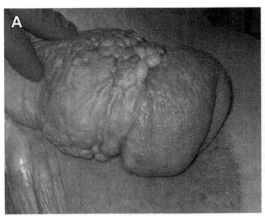
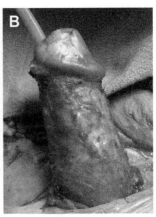

Fig. 9. (*A*) Patient who underwent meshed split-thickness skin graft to the proximal penile shaft after necrotizing genital infection debridement. The distal shaft skin was left in place, later becoming grossly lymphedematous and enveloping the glans. (*B*) Same patient after resection of all grafted and native penile skin.

the glans. However, efforts to treat benign and malignant disease in an organ-preserving manner have led to techniques such as glans resurfacing.[29] This technique involves removing glans skin and replacing it with a split-thickness skin graft[30] or by grafting onto the ends of the corporal bodies after distal penectomy to recreate the appearance of the glans (see **Fig. 3**).[31]

Surgeons have tried to prevent nocturnal erections, a normal occurrence during the rapid-eye movement sleep cycle, after urologic surgery for decades. However, there is little evidence to support success of medical therapies to prevent erections.[32] This reemphasizes the need to closely affix the graft to the penis and use a dressing that prevents shear.

SUMMARY

Many disease processes may result in a need for replacement of penile skin. Thick split-thickness grafts are the most appropriate choice for penile skin reconstruction because of the special characteristics of penile skin, namely thin, hairless skin, with stretch capability. Reconstruction of the penile skin can be challenging because of the expanding nature of the penis and difficult contours of the area. Using proper surgical technique and postoperative wound care maximizes graft success.

REFERENCES

1. Proksch E, Brandner JM, Jensen JM. The skin: an indispensable barrier. Exp Dermatol 2008;17(12): 1063–72.
2. Taylor GI, Gianoutsos MP, Morris SF. The neurovascular territories of the skin and muscles: anatomic study and clinical implications. Plast Reconstr Surg 1994;94(1):1–36.
3. Corps BV. The effect of graft thickness, donor site and graft bed on graft shrinkage in the hooded rat. Br J Plast Surg 1969;22(2):125–33.
4. Shuster S, Black MM, McVitie E. The influence of age and sex on skin thickness, skin collagen and density. Br J Dermatol 1975;93(6):639–43.
5. Garaffa G, Christopher N, Ralph DJ. The management of genital lymphoedema. BJU Int 2008; 102(4):480–4.
6. Morey AF, Meng MV, McAninch JW. Skin graft reconstruction of chronic genital lymphedema. Urology 1997;50(3):423–6.
7. Tang SH, Kamat D, Santucci RA. Modern management of adult-acquired buried penis. Urology 2008; 72(1):124–7.
8. Bracka A. Hypospadias repair: the two-stage alternative. Br J Urol 1995;76(Suppl 3):31–41.
9. Schreiter F, Noll F. Mesh graft urethroplasty using split thickness skin graft or foreskin. J Urol 1989; 142(5):1223–6.
10. Converse JM, Uhlschmid GK, Ballantyne DL Jr. "Plasmatic circulation" in skin grafts. The phase of serum imbibition. Plast Reconstr Surg 1969;43(5): 495–9.
11. Clemmesen T. The early circulation in split skin grafts. Acta Chir Scand 1962;124:11.
12. Eriksson G, Klingenstrom P, Nylen B, et al. Electron microscopic studies on the epidermis in human split-skin autografts. Scand J Plast Reconstr Surg 1968;2(2):83–90.
13. Converse JM, Smahel J, Ballantyne DL Jr, et al. Inosculation of vessels of skin graft and host bed: a fortuitous encounter. Br J Plast Surg 1975;28(4): 274–82.
14. Ponten B. Grafted skin. Acta Chir Scand Suppl 1960;(Suppl 257):1–78.

15. Smahel J. The healing of skin grafts. Clin Plast Surg 1977;4(3):409–24.
16. Waris T, Astrand K, Hamalainen H, et al. Regeneration of cold, warmth and heat-pain sensibility in human skin grafts. Br J Plast Surg 1989;42(5):576–80.
17. Flowers RS. Unexpected postoperative problems in skin grafting. Surg Clin North Am 1970;50(2):439–56.
18. Perry AW, Sutkin HS, Gottlieb LJ, et al. Skin graft survival–the bacterial answer. Ann Plast Surg 1989;22(6):479–83.
19. Jabs AD Jr, Wider TM, DeBellis J, et al. The effect of fibrin glue on skin grafts in infected sites. Plast Reconstr Surg 1992;89(2):268–71.
20. McDougal WS. Lymphedema of the external genitalia. J Urol 2003;170(3):711–6.
21. Saltz R, Dimick A, Harris C, et al. Application of autologous fibrin glue in burn wounds. J Burn Care Rehabil 1989;10(6):504–7.
22. Vedung S, Hedlung A. Fibrin glue: its use for skin grafting of contaminated burn wounds in areas difficult to immobilize. J Burn Care Rehabil 1993;14(3):356–8.
23. Morris MS, Morey AF, Stackhouse DA, et al. Fibrin sealant as tissue glue: preliminary experience in complex genital reconstructive surgery. Urology 2006;67(4):688–91 [discussion: 691–2].
24. Malone PR, Thomas JS, Blick C. A tie-over dressing for graft application in distal penectomy and glans resurfacing: the TODGA technique. BJU Int 201 107(5):836–40.
25. Schneider AM, Morykwas MJ, Argenta LC. A ne and reliable method of securing skin grafts to th difficult recipient bed. Plast Reconstr Surg 1998 102(4):1195–8.
26. Blackburn JH 2nd, Boemi L, Hall WW, et al. Nega tive-pressure dressings as a bolster for skin graft Ann Plast Surg 1998;40(5):453–7.
27. Weinfeld AB, Kelley P, Yuksel E, et al. Circumferer tial negative-pressure dressing (VAC) to bolste skin grafts in the reconstruction of the penile sha and scrotum. Ann Plast Surg 2005;54(2):178–83.
28. Brady SC, Snelling CF, Chow G. Comparison of donc site dressings. Ann Plast Surg 1980;5(3):238–43.
29. Depasquale I, Park AJ, Bracka A. The treatment c balanitis xerotica obliterans. BJU Int 2000;86(4 459–65.
30. Bracka A. Glans resection and plastic repair. BJU Ir 2010;105(1):136–44.
31. Palminteri E, Berdondini E, Lazzeri M, et al. Resu facing and reconstruction of the glans penis. Eu Urol 2007;52(3):893–8.
32. DeCastro BJ, Costabile RA, McMann LP, et al. Ora ketoconazole for prevention of postoperative penile erection: a placebo controlled, randomized double-blind trial. J Urol 2008;179(5):1930–2.

ndex

Urol Clin N Am 40 (2013) 449–455
http://dx.doi.org/10.1016/S0094-0143(13)00057-8
0094-0143/13/$ – see front matter © 2013 Elsevier Inc. All rights reserved.

Moving?

Make sure your subscription moves with you!

To notify us of your new address, find your **Clinics Account Number** (located on your mailing label above your name), and contact customer service at:

Email: journalscustomerservice-usa@elsevier.com

800-654-2452 (subscribers in the U.S. & Canada)
314-447-8871 (subscribers outside of the U.S. & Canada)

Fax number: 314-447-8029

Elsevier Health Sciences Division
Subscription Customer Service
3251 Riverport Lane
Maryland Heights, MO 63043

*To ensure uninterrupted delivery of your subscription, please notify us at least 4 weeks in advance of move.

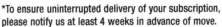

Printed and bound by CPI Group (UK) Ltd, Croydon, CR0 4YY

03/10/2024

01040301-0012